A Practical Guide to
Self-Massage

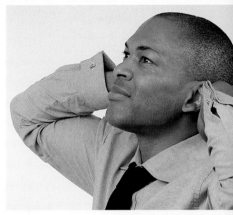

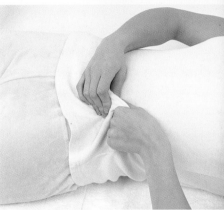

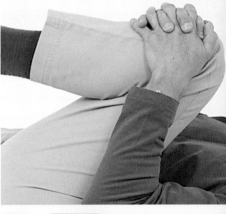

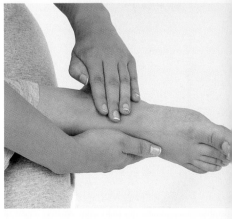

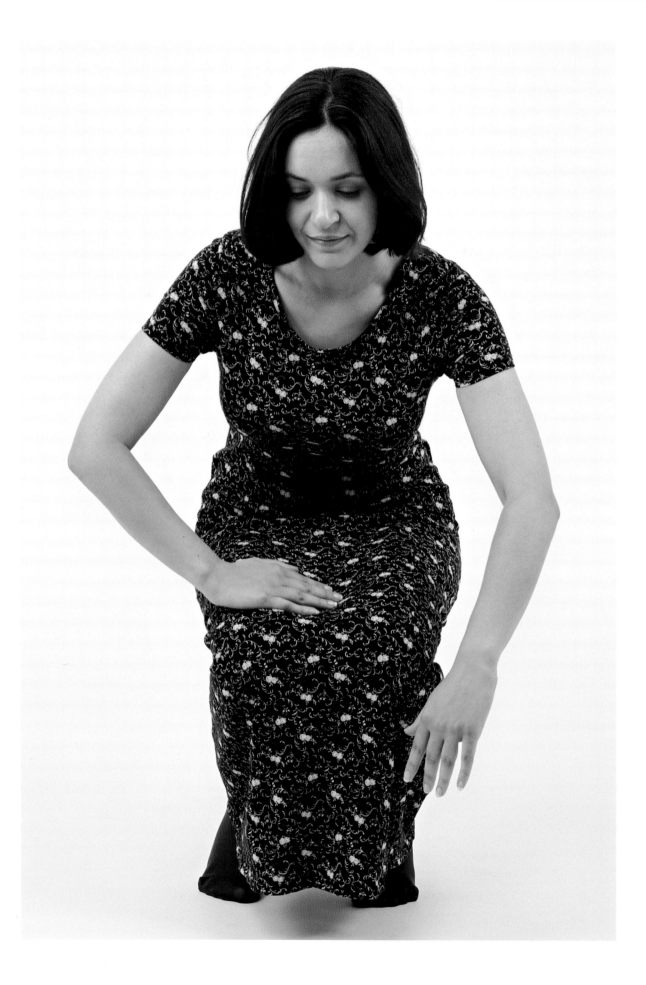

A Practical Guide to
Self-Massage

Over 50 Simple Exercises and Relaxation Techniques to Improve Your Health and Well-Being

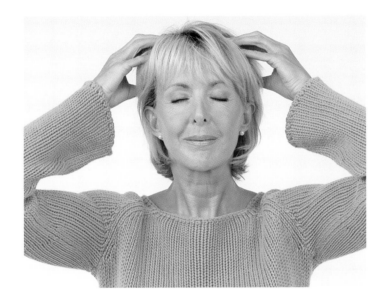

MARY ATKINSON

Reader's Digest

The Reader's Digest Association, Inc.
Pleasantville, New York/Montreal/London/Hong Kong

◆

To my father, Reg Peplow

◆

A READER'S DIGEST BOOK

This edition published by The Reader's Digest Association
by arrangement with Cico Books

FOR CICO BOOKS
Project Editor: Richard Emerson
Designer: David Fordham
Photographer: Geoff Dann

FOR READER'S DIGEST
U.S. Project Editor: Barbara Booth
Canadian Project Editor: Pamela Johnson
Editorial Consultant: Ruth Oppenheimer, PT
Project Designer: George McKeon
Executive Editor, Trade Publishing: Dolores York
Vice President & Publisher, Trade Publishing: Harold Clarke

Library of Congress Cataloging-in-Publication Data

Atkinson, Mary, 1954-
   A practical guide to self-massage for health & vitality / Mary Atkinson.
      p. cm.
   Includes index.
   ISBN 0-7621-0571-2
   1. Massage. 2. Self-care, Health. I. Title: Self massage for health & vitality. II. Title

RA780.5.A85 2006
615.8'22—dc22

                                                                                    2005050198

Address any comments to:
   The Reader's Digest Association, Inc.
   Adult Trade Publishing
   Reader's Digest Road
   Pleasantville, NY 10570-7000

Note to Our Readers

   The information in this book should not be substituted for, or used to alter, medical therapy without your doctor's advice. If you have a history of congestive heart failure, blood clots, cancer, lymphedema, or other specific health problems, consult your physician for guidance before doing any of the exercises in this book.

For more Reader's Digest products and information, visit our website:
www.rd.com (in the United States)
www.rd.ca (in Canada)
www.readersdigest.com.au (in Australia)
www.rdasia.com (in Asia)
www.readersdigest.co.uk (in the UK)

Printed in Singapore

10 9 8 7 6 5 4 3 2 (hardcover)

Contents

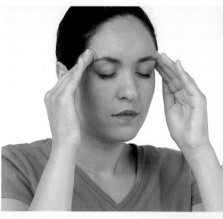

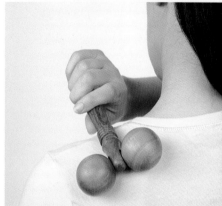

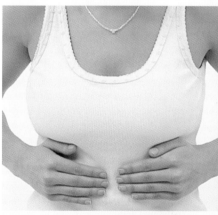

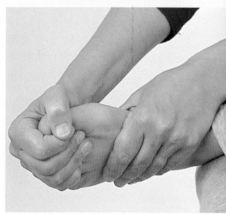

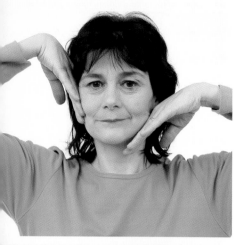

4 AT HOME 56

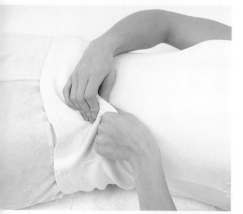

5 ON THE MOVE 92

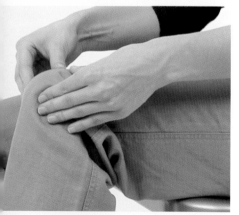

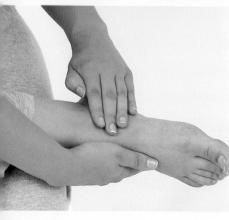

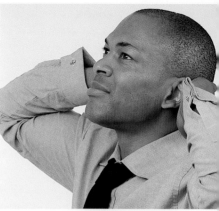

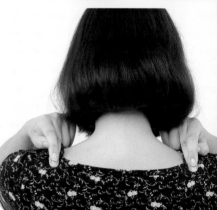

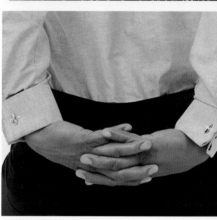

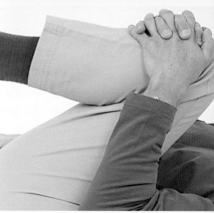

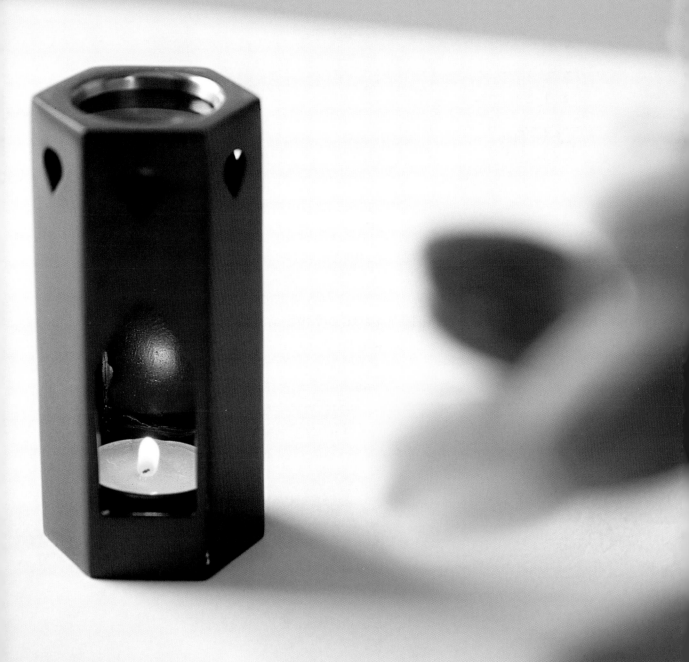

1 SELF-MASSAGE: THE BASICS AND BENEFITS

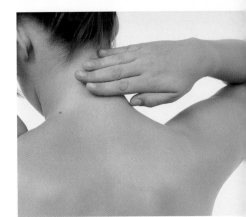

The joy of self-massage is that you can use it whenever you need to. Self-massage can help alleviate pain and stiffness while you are sitting at your desk, calm your nerves before an important event, boost your energy levels, or warm your toes on a cold evening. It is all in your own hands. You can pinpoint the exact location of those trouble spots and use the right amount of pressure. So make use of these techniques and tips in your daily life. As you begin to reap the benefits, you will wonder how you ever managed before you mastered the art of self-massage.

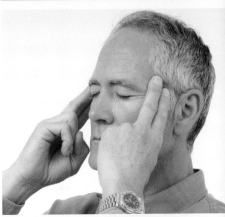

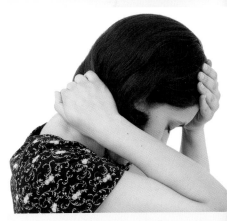

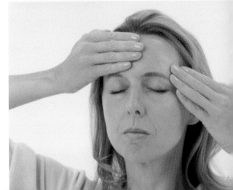

Welcome to self-massage

This book is for people who lead busy, stressful lives, and that probably refers to most of us. It offers practical, easy-to-follow advice for relieving symptoms of minor health complaints.

Self-massage does not preclude the advice of a health professional. If you're concerned about your health, talk to your physician before attempting any of these exercises.

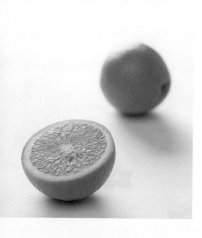

Over the following pages, you will discover how learning a few basic self-massage strokes can be a major step toward achieving and maintaining good health and vitality. The book is divided into two parts. The first chapters offer the knowledge necessary to help you appreciate the therapeutic powers of self-massage and the role it can play in your daily life.

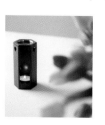

Chapter 1 outlines both the physical and psychological benefits of massage. It explores the development of one of the oldest forms of healing arts and discusses how massage has now become a well-established antidote to the pressures and demands of modern living. This chapter offers a brief introduction to the effect of stress on health and to the different bodily systems, thus providing a better understanding of the ways in which self-massage can relax or invigorate mind and body.

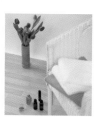

Chapter 2 highlights safety guidelines for self-massage. And while all you really need to massage yourself to better health is a pair of hands and your natural ability, this chapter also offers advice on maximizing its benefits by using carrier oils, aromatic oils, and massage tools.

Chapter 3 shows you how to practice the various self-massage techniques that are used later in the book. These include movements drawn from different cultures and range from passive holding techniques to more vigorous beating and the use of

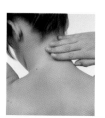

acupressure. Each technique is explored in detail with illustrated instructions showing how, where, and when to use it to derive optimum benefits.

The next chapters take you through a variety of self-help sequences and programs to help you deal with common ailments and maintain good health and well-being. There are lifestyle tips, such as dietary ideas and postural advice, to

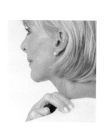

complement the massage movements.

Chapter 4 looks at those routines that can be enjoyed in the comfort of your own home —whether lying in bed, watching TV, or relaxing in a comfortable chair. These sequences help ease constipation, cope with premenstrual tension, and boost your immune system.

Chapter 5 describes self-massage routines to use while on 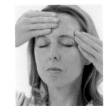 the move—whether on a bus, in an airplane, or in a shopping mall—and shows how to overcome common ailments such as cramps and sinus congestion, as well as dealing with jet lag, anxiety, and cold hands.

Work-related ailments are the focus of Chapter 6 with routines designed to help with problems such as repetitive strain injury, eye strain, and tension headaches. These simple routines can be performed during work breaks or at the start or end of a long work day.

Chapter 7 concludes the book with 10 different programs to revitalize, relax, and boost general health and fitness. Simply choose the routines that suit your personal lifestyle and needs—and then plan ways to fit them into your daily or weekly routine.

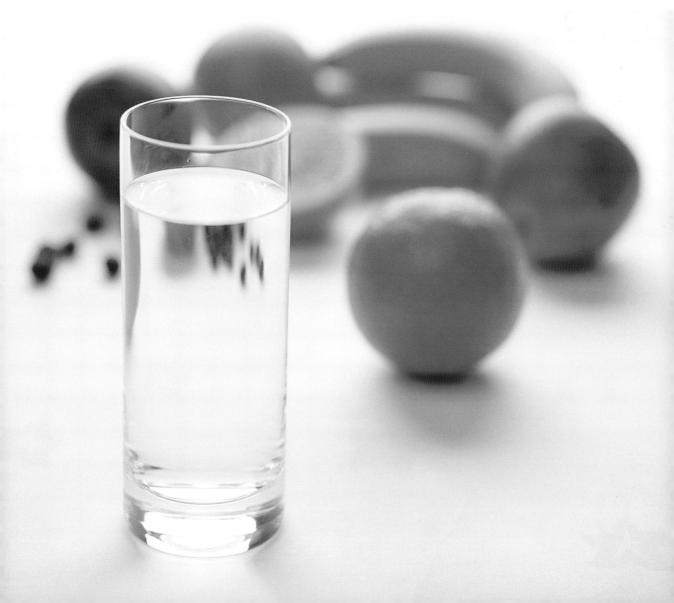

Massage—an ancient art

Massage is one of the oldest forms of healing. Its history in China and India can be traced back thousands of years. Today massage is enjoyed by people of all ages and walks of life. Techniques from different cultures are incorporated into massage routines that provide effective treatment for common ailments associated with our modern, stressful lifestyles.

Eastern massage

Among the earliest records of the therapeutic use of massage are ancient Chinese books, dated around 3000 B.C. The Chinese were particularly interested in studying the effects of pressure when applied to different parts of the body. Over time they developed techniques, known as amma, using pressure at specific points to help the body heal itself. It was from these early discoveries that simple forms of acupuncture and acupressure were developed.

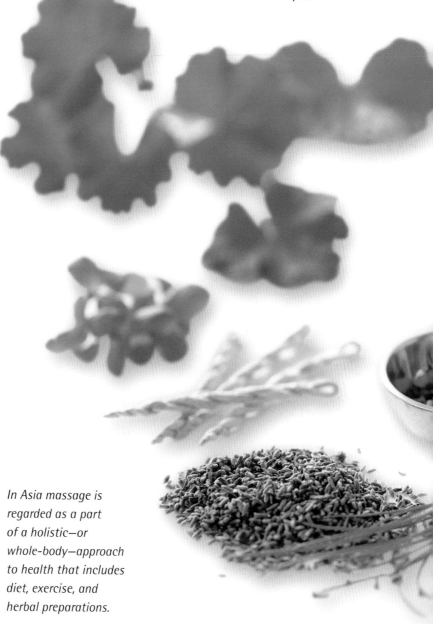

In Asia massage is regarded as a part of a holistic—or whole-body—approach to health that includes diet, exercise, and herbal preparations.

In India massage has long been an integral part of daily life. Ancient Hindu texts, dating back to 1800 B.C., teach a complete healing system based on a truly holistic approach to health, advocating the use of diet, yoga, massage, breathing exercises, and purifying techniques to promote health and prevent illness. This traditional system of medicine, known as Ayurveda, which means the "science of life," is still widely practiced in India today. A daily self-massage, called abhyanga, uses natural vegetable oils and is one of the recommendations for promoting strength and flexibility, improving skin texture, and boosting the immune system.

Western massage

Massage has had a more checkered history in the West. Interest was strong around 500 B.C. when the Greeks embraced it as

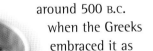

part of their rigorous health-and-fitness regimens. The Greek physician, Hippocrates, known as the "Father of Medicine," was an enthusiastic advocate of the health benefits of massage and argued, all those years ago, that doctors should be trained to massage: "The physician must be experienced in many things but assuredly rubbing."

The Romans had the same passion for massage as the Greeks. Roman masters invested their time in bathing, exercise, and massage, not only to maintain good health but also to treat common ailments. Indeed, records show that Julius Caesar was rubbed and pinched all over every day to help relieve his neuralgia. Gladiators used massage to enhance their prowess in sporting events, and soldiers believed squeezing, pinching, and pummeling helped them in battle—and afterward, too, to relieve pain and promote recovery.

With the decline of the Roman Empire, massage fell from favor in the West. But in the sixteenth century, enlightened physicians once again took an interest in the therapeutic benefits of massage and incorporated various techniques into their medical treatments.

As knowledge of anatomy and physiology increased, so, too, did the use of massage for treating diseases and ailments. In the early nineteenth century, a Swedish physiologist, Per Henrick Ling, introduced a system of exercises and massage movements that later developed into the treatment now called physical therapy.

In the 1870's the news of the benefits of massage spread to the United States, and 1884 saw the first book on massage published here. During the First World War, massage was used to provide pain relief and treatment for injured soldiers suffering from nerve damage and shell shock.

Massage today

However, the tremendous boom in technology in the West in the 1940's and '50's overshadowed the benefits of holistic forms of treatment such as massage, and once again these "physical therapies" declined in popularity. Thankfully, increasing demand for natural ways of promoting health and well-being has brought an awareness of the wonderfully beneficial effects of massage, and self-massage has re-emerged as an important form of health care.

Massage is now established as an antidote to the demands of modern life and is taken into homes, offices, schools, hospitals, and even airports to reduce tension, ease anxiety, increase clarity of thought, and promote positive health and well-being.

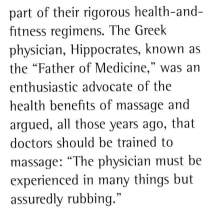

Benefits of self-massage

Self-massage can help bring instant relief from everyday ailments. And since the benefits are cumulative, it offers many long-term advantages, such as helping to boost and maintain positive health and mental well-being.

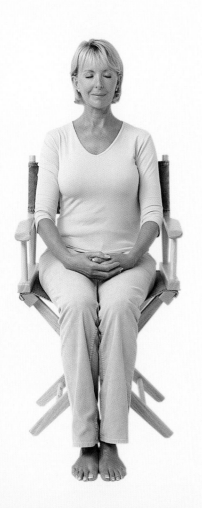

Massage can offer far-reaching benefits for both mind and body. Increasingly, this fact is being acknowledged by many employers who are following the Oriental tradition of introducing massage into the workplace to boost performance and production, and to reduce levels of sick leave among employees suffering stress-related health complaints.

Massage is the manipulation of the body's soft tissue—skin, fat, muscle—and the connective tissue that holds organs and underlying structures in place. It involves a series of movements, mainly using the hands. Each movement is applied in a particular way in order to have a specific effect. Brisk early-morning massage, for example, awakens and refreshes you from head to toe. Gentle massage in the evening prepares you for a deep restorative sleep.

Tailor to your needs

Massage affects the circulation of blood and lymph, as well as the muscles, nerves, and digestion. And since mind and body are intertwined, imbalance in one system influences overall physical and emotional well-being. As you begin to appreciate the effects of different massage movements on all the structures and systems of the body, you will be able to adapt your techniques to ensure that your massage provides the benefits you seek.

MASSAGE BENEFITS IN BRIEF

◆ Self-massage can target trouble spots, especially in the muscles and joints, and helps relieve localized areas of pain, thus easing symptoms of tension such as eye strain, sore feet, headache, and backache.

◆ Regular self-massage helps promote the strength and flexibility of the muscles and joints, improving mobility and helping to prevent the aches, pains, and stiffness associated with everyday life.

◆ Brisk self-massage movements increase physical and mental energy levels, encouraging a feeling of "get up and go" and mental alertness.

◆ Soothing self-massage movements produce a general state of relaxation of mind and body, thus easing tension and anxiety, alleviating the cumulative effects of stress, and encouraging the body to function more effectively.

◆ Relaxing self-massage encourages a better quality of sleep, which in turn leads to

Creating a relaxing atmosphere with candles and fragrant oils enhances the relaxing effects of a self-massage routine.

improved temperament and general health and well-being.

◆ Stimulating self-massage boosts blood flow around the body, ensuring a steady supply of oxygen and nutrients to the tissues and generating heat to warm areas, such as hands and feet, that are prone to cold.

◆ Rhythmical self-massage aids the removal of waste products and toxins from the body and helps prevent a buildup of these impurities, which can lead to muscle pain, headaches, dull skin, sinus congestion, and fatigue.

◆ Massage movements can be effective in removing excess fluid from the body, thus reducing puffiness, especially in the ankles and feet.

◆ Self-massage boosts the immune system, helping to prevent and fight infections.

◆ Self-massage brings increased self-awareness, which often leads to early recognition of stress signals—both physical and psychological—and an understanding of the need to incorporate regular relaxation sessions in everyday life.

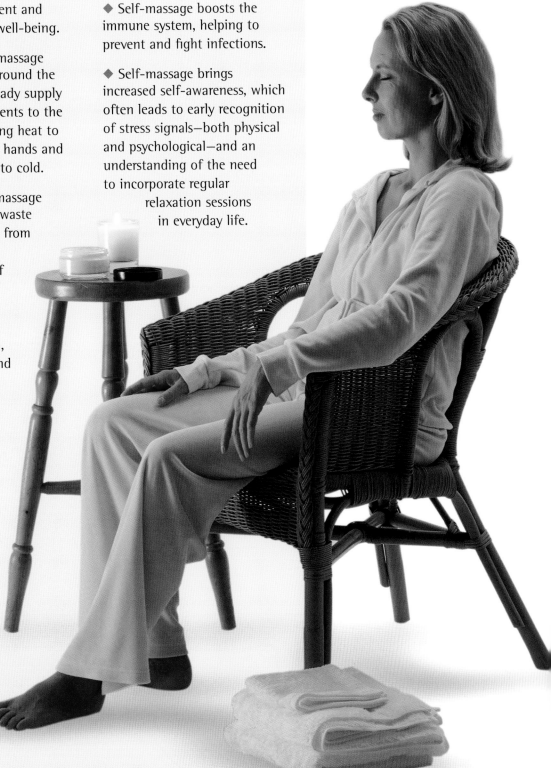

Self-massage for today's stress

Our lives today are so stressful that we cannot even try to avoid the many factors that cause our blood pressure to rise, our muscles to tense, and our heart rates to race. So the best approach is to introduce strategies for managing stress more effectively.

Self-massage is particularly beneficial for inducing physical and mental relaxation and offers a simple and effective way to cope with those everyday pressures that send stress levels soaring.

Stress is a natural response to any kind of extra demand, pressure, or change—pleasant or unpleasant, real or perceived —that is placed on the mind or body. Stress can be positive. A healthy level of stress creates the motivation to complete important tasks, give the competitive edge at business meetings and sporting events, and provide exhilaration before an exciting event.

Stress thresholds

Stress becomes harmful only when we lose the ability to deal in a calm and rational way with the extra demands placed on us. In other words, there is an imbalance in the level of stress and our ability to cope with it. It is a very personal reaction. Everyone has a different stress threshold. What seems invigorating and

challenging to one person at a certain time may cause anxiety to another in a different situation. This can vary from day to day according to circumstances.

Managing stress

Stress management involves recognizing and controlling the demands placed on you and being positive and realistic about your ability to cope with them. Stress has a cumulative effect. Unless we find ways of reducing it, problems get even more daunting and threatening, which increases the stress—and so the spiral continues.

Mental and emotional health are directly linked, with physical tension and illness combining to exacerbate the problem. And if you have any doubts about this connection, think how often anxiety over

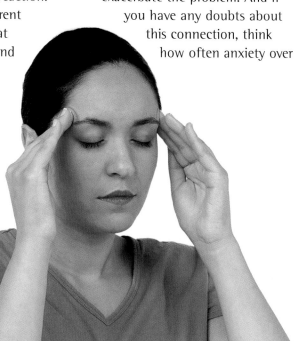

At times of stress, rubbing the temples using slow, circular movements can calm nerves and ease the spirit.

a family argument, or a visit to the orthodontist, have manifested as headaches or stomach cramps, making the situation worse. Similarly, recovery from the physical symptoms of an illness can be aided or hindered by your mental or emotional state.

"A mind refreshed"

The beneficial effects of massage on physical ailments have been documented for thousands of years, but it is only in fairly recent times that massage techniques were shown to calm and settle a stressed and troubled mind. An eminent nineteenth-century physician, Dr. Stretch Dowse, wrote in 1887: "The mind, which before massage is in a perturbed, restless, vacillating, and even despondent state, becomes after massage, calm, quiet, peaceful, and subdued; in fact, the wearied and worried mind had been converted into a mind restful, placid, and refreshed."

One of the joys of self-massage is that it can aid you on a physical and psychological level. As aches and pains are rubbed away by your massage movements, you feel calmer and more able to cope with daily pressures in a relaxed and positive frame of mind.

Many research studies are exploring the therapeutic effects of massage on the physiological and

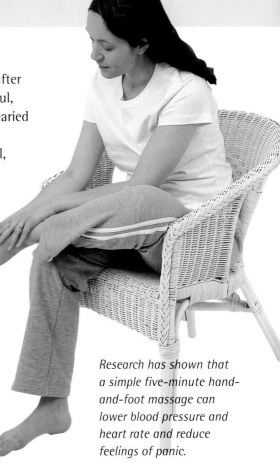

Research has shown that a simple five-minute hand-and-foot massage can lower blood pressure and heart rate and reduce feelings of panic.

STRESS FACTS

◆ Medical experts say stress may be responsible for up to 75 percent of all diseases in the Western world, ranging from skin disorders such as psoriasis and eczema through headaches, digestive illnesses, backache, muscle tension, and depression to potentially life-threatening conditions, including obesity, alcoholism, high blood pressure, heart disease, and stroke.

◆ A study at the Touch Research Institute in Miami, Florida, used physical and emotional assessment methods to compare stress levels of two groups of adults over a five-week period. One group received a regular massage, while the other did not. Findings showed that massage has a positive effect in helping to increase relaxation, reduce anxiety, and enhance mental alertness.

psychological aspects of stress. Studies that have been completed so far (see left) conclude that massage has an important role to play in the alleviation of stress and stress-related illnesses.

In the hustle and bustle of daily activities, we often deprive ourselves of the opportunity to be still and quiet and to simply "be ourselves." Finding time in the day to give yourself a massage, if only for five minutes, can provide an incentive to switch off from spiraling worries and daily hassles, allowing space for mind and body to relax and recharge, ready to face the world again.

How stress affects you

Short bouts of stress can have a beneficial effect, increasing energy levels and mental alertness. But over a prolonged period, stress puts both mind and body in a constant state of "overdrive" that saps mental and physical energy.

The effects are cumulative and can creep up so slowly that many people hardly notice the changes occurring within themselves until they begin to suffer symptoms.

In any stressful situation, the body responds by tensing the muscles and releasing hormones such as cortisol and epinephrine to prepare for instant action. This is known as the "fight or flight" response and is a survival tactic intended to cope with a purely physical threat, such as escaping from a blazing building.

As you can see from the diagram opposite, the short-term effects of the "fight or flight" response are designed to promote rapid action in a crisis. Normal functions are restored once the threat is over and physical activity, whether in dealing with the threat or fleeing from it, has utilized the increased energy

supplies. However, stress today is more often psychological—arising from work, money, or relationship problems, for example—yet the body still reacts as if a physical response is required.

Our more sedentary lifestyles in the Western world mean that we may have little physical outlet for the stress response, so the stress hormones build up and we live under a perpetual low level of "crisis" for many days, months, and even years.

Over a longer period of time, physical and mental health can become seriously affected, mainly because the stress hormones impede major bodily systems, such as circulation and immunity.

STRESS TIPS AND TECHNIQUES

There are various relaxation techniques you can combine with self-massage to help you manage stress. Try to find a few methods that work for you and set aside some "me time" each day to practice them. As you get more proficient, you can use them any time you feel tense.

◆ DEEP BREATHING: Breathe in very slowly, taking the air deep into your lungs. Watch your abdomen rise. Hold for a count of 3. Breathe out. Repeat as often as you wish. Feel the tension ease with every breath.

◆ COUNTING MEDITATION: Find a comfortable position. Close your eyes. Slowly count to 10. Then start at 1 again. Clear your mind of everything but counting. If anything intrudes into your thoughts, acknowledge it, release it. Carry on counting.

◆ VISUALIZATION: Close your eyes and imagine a relaxing scene you know very well—a secluded beach, a tranquil wood, or a favorite room, for example. Focus on every detail—sights, sounds, smells—until you can almost believe you're there.

Hormones

SHORT-TERM: The pituitary gland activates other glands to release hormones that prepare the body for instant action.
LONG-TERM: Stress hormones depress the immune system, leading to increased risk of disease.

Mood

SHORT-TERM: Need for increased concentration.
LONG-TERM: Anxiety, depression.

(3) Heart

SHORT-TERM: Beats strongly to pump extra blood to the muscles and brain.
LONG-TERM: Risk of chest pains and high blood pressure, palpitations.

(5) Liver

SHORT-TERM: Releases extra supplies of glucose and fats into bloodstream for energy.
LONG-TERM: Risk of permanently raised levels of sugars and fats leading to heart disease, stroke, and diabetes.

(7) Bowels and bladder

SHORT-TERM: Urge to empty to make body as light as possible for action.
LONG-TERM: Diarrhea, constipation, frequent urge to urinate, irritable bowel syndrome.

Muscles

SHORT-TERM: Tense to ensure optimum performance, either in facing the attacker or making an instant getaway.
LONG-TERM: Achiness, stiffness, muscle spasms.

Brain (1)

SHORT-TERM: Increased blood supplies initially promote alertness and clarity of thought.
LONG-TERM: Tension headaches and migraines, nervousness, hesitancy, lack of confidence.

Saliva (2)

SHORT-TERM: Dries up because eating is not a necessity right now.
LONG-TERM: Dry mouth and lump-in-the-throat sensation.

Lungs (4)

SHORT-TERM: Breathing rate increases to take in oxygen to fuel muscles and brain.
LONG-TERM: Cough, shortness of breath, hyperventilation.

Stomach (6)

SHORT-TERM: Digestive enzymes inhibited, increased stomach acid levels.
LONG-TERM: Heartburn, indigestion, gastric ulcers.

Sexual organs (8)

SHORT-TERM: Blood is diverted away because sexual activity is not a priority.
LONG-TERM: Loss of interest in sex, impotence in men, women's inability to reach orgasm, menstrual disorders.

Skin

SHORT-TERM: Becomes pale, dry and sensitive as blood is diverted from the skin to other parts of the body.
LONG-TERM: Dry-skin conditions, itching, eczema, rashes.

Systems—blood circulation

Every cell requires a constant supply of oxygen and fuel, such as glucose, as well as the rapid removal of toxic wastes produced by all the normal chemical processes occurring in the tissues. But this supply can be impeded by poor posture, illness, and lack of physical activity. Self-massage can play a part in restoring a healthy blood circulation and thus help to maintain health and vitality.

Proper blood circulation is essential to the health and vitality of all bodily systems. The driving force for the circulation is the heart, a muscular bag that pumps the blood along a continuous figure-eight circuit, traveling between the lungs, the heart, and the tissues of the body (see right).

Outward path

On the first stage of its journey, blood collects oxygen from the lungs and surges from the heart under great pressure, on the way to collecting nutrients such as glucose, fats, and amino acids from the liver and digestive tract.

The blood is carried in arteries, which are blood vessels with thick muscular walls that widen and narrow again as blood pumps through them, creating the "pulse beat" we can detect in the wrist, upper thigh, and neck.

The arteries form a network of tubes reaching all body regions. These blood vessels branch off into increasingly smaller tubes, called arterioles, and then into tiny capillaries, which carry oxygen and nutrients to individual cells.

Return path

On the journey back to the heart, blood collects the wasted gases and other unwanted products that have drained out of the cells into the capillaries and then into larger venules. It then passes into large blood vessels—the veins.

The blood is now under far less pressure than in the arterial system, so the vein walls are much thinner. Many veins have nonreturn valves to prevent a backflow of blood. If the valves stop working, blood may collect in the legs, causing the veins to swell and protrude—a condition known as varicose veins.

The cells need rich supplies of oxygen and nutrients to function at their optimum level. If the circulation is sluggish or impaired, the cells are not only starved of nourishment but stagnant wastes begin to build up in the tissues.

As a result, energy levels may plummet; muscles can feel stiff, painful, and tired; the brain starts to suffer lapses in concentration and memory; the hair looks lackluster; and the skin takes on a dull and tired appearance.

Hormones

The blood collects hormones from the endocrine glands, where they are produced, and takes them to target organs, where they trigger a reaction.

(2) Heart

The heart is divided into four chambers—two atria and two ventricles—that pump in sequence to maintain the circulation.

(4) Liver

The liver is well supplied with blood vessels, allowing the blood to collect stores of nutrients, such as glucose and other important chemicals, and distribute them throughout the body.

(6) Digestive tract

Blood vessels in the digestive tract collect minerals, vitamins, glucose, fats, and amino acids (building blocks of proteins) and deliver these nutrients to the cells, providing energy and raw materials for their chemical activities.

Muscles

To operate efficiently and prevent fatigue and cramp, the muscles rely on a healthy circulation for a constant supply of nutrients and speedy removal of wastes.

Brain (1)

The blood supplies the brain with glucose—the only fuel it can use—and oxygen. A healthy circulation boosts concentration, alertness, and memory.

Lungs (3)

Healthy lungs ensure that the blood is richly supplied with energy-giving oxygen and that carbon dioxide is speedily removed.

Kidneys (5)

The kidneys play a vital role in the circulation of the blood by maintaining optimum fluid levels and filtering out impurities.

Immune system

The blood carries immune-system cells, known as leukocytes, and special protein molecules called antibodies that attack and destroy bacteria and viruses and also help guard against repeat infection.

Skin

A rich blood supply to surface tissues keeps skin and hair in good condition; it also ensures that impurities are removed through perspiration.

Systems—muscles and joints

The body is capable of a wide range of movements. This flexibility is due to a complex system of bones, muscles, and connective tissues.

Self-massage promotes the health, strength, and flexibility of the muscles. As the Greek physician Hippocrates wrote in 400 B.C., "Rubbing can bind a joint that is too loose and also loosen a joint that is too hard."

Bones form the basic framework of the body. Where movable bones meet, they form joints. Different types of joints allow varying degrees of movement. This movement is facilitated by voluntary muscles—that is, the ones we consciously control to bring about movement, whether raising an arm or lifting an eyelid.

There are about 650 voluntary muscles in the body. Most are attached to bones on either side of a joint by cords of connective tissue called tendons. A muscle pulls on a tendon, which moves the bone, causing a leg to be bent, for example. Muscles work in pairs. One contracts to move a bone; the other relaxes to allow the movement—and vice versa.

Muscles have their own supply of blood and lymphatic vessels. As muscle fibers relax, blood flows in, bringing fresh supplies of oxygen and nutrients needed for muscles to generate energy and heat. As fibers contract, blood is forced out, taking with it any impurities and by-products of chemical processes.

If muscles work so vigorously that oxygen is used up quicker than the body can deliver it, a waste product—lactic acid—is produced, leading to fatigue, soreness, discomfort, and pain.

Some muscle fibers are always partially contracted, even when not actively being used, in order to maintain posture—whether sitting, standing, or lying down.

Muscle constriction

If muscles are held abnormally contracted for a long time, owing to poor postural habits, stress, or sitting for extended periods in front of a computer screen, it can cause muscle tension. The flow of blood and lymph is impeded, muscle fibers are deprived of their full quota of oxygen and nutrients, and toxic wastes accumulate and stagnate.

Over time the muscle tissue changes in structure, which may be felt as hard lumps or nodules under the skin. This is most apparent in the muscles of the shoulder and upper back. Muscle tension can build up so slowly that we may not notice it until we feel discomfort, soreness, stiffness, and aches and pains.

MUSCLES AND JOINTS: BENEFITS OF SELF-MASSAGE

Self-massage benefits muscles and joints by easing tension, relieving constriction, and thus aiding mobility.

◆ As muscles are encouraged to relax, this brings a greater awareness of the muscular tension that is being stored in our bodies by everyday activities.

◆ Muscle fibers are stretched, broadened, and separated, and any adhesions are broken down, enabling muscles to contract and relax more efficiently.

◆ The increased flow of blood and lymph brings fresh supplies of nutrients and oxygen to muscles and joints and removes waste products and excess fluid. This helps improve joint mobility and reduces the stiffness, aches, and tiredness so often associated with long periods of standing or repetitive hand movements.

◆ Increased blood supply and frictional heat create warmth in the area, which encourages relaxation and natural pain relief, aiding the recovery of muscle soreness after physical activity.

◆ Facial massage relaxes the muscles, which helps erase fine tension lines and tones the muscles to give a younger, fresher appearance to the complexion.

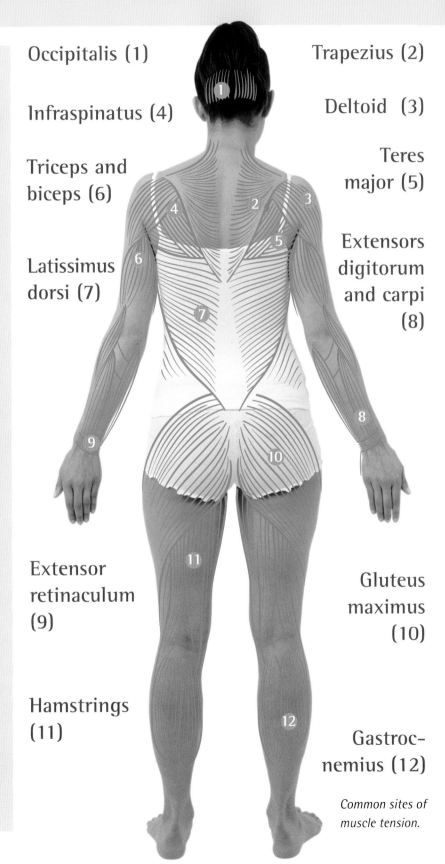

Occipitalis (1)

Trapezius (2)

Infraspinatus (4)

Deltoid (3)

Triceps and biceps (6)

Teres major (5)

Latissimus dorsi (7)

Extensors digitorum and carpi (8)

Extensor retinaculum (9)

Gluteus maximus (10)

Hamstrings (11)

Gastroc-nemius (12)

Common sites of muscle tension.

Systems—the lymphatics

The lymphatics are a network of fluid-filled tubes and specialized organs and tissues. Often disregarded, they play a vital role in the drainage of excess fluids from the tissues, the collection of fats and proteins, and the defense of the body from disease organisms.

Self-massage can play an important role in keeping the lymphatic system working efficiently.

The blood circulation is assisted by the lymphatic system, a highly efficient cleansing and defense system that extends throughout the body via an intricate network of nodes, vessels, and tubes.

The lymphatic system has many vital functions. It drains excess fluid and removes waste products from the tissue spaces, collects protein from the cells, absorbs fats from the intestines, removes potentially pathogenic (harmful) organisms such as viruses and bacteria and carries them to the lymph nodes, where they can be destroyed by white blood cells, and produces antibodies needed to provide immunity to disease.

Cell drainage

The lymphatic system is filled with a fluid called lymph. The primary job of the lymphatics is to act as the body's drainage system, removing excess fluid and impurities from the tissues.

On its journey, lymph passes through lymph nodes (sometimes known as "glands") that are placed at strategic positions along the network, including in the head, face, and neck, under the armpits, in the crook of the elbow, behind the knees, and in the groin and intestines, close to the most likely areas of infection.

Lymph nodes act as filters to cleanse the lymph and remove potentially harmful organisms before the fluid eventually drains into the venous circulation at a site called the thoracic duct.

Disease prevention

Special white blood cells known as leukocytes, produced in the bone marrow and spleen, are stored in the lymph nodes and other tissues ready to fight infection. Whenever there is a threat of invasion by disease organisms, the immune cells in the nearest lymph nodes divide to produce extra "soldier" cells to repel the invaders.

Some cells produce antibodies that attach to disease organisms, preventing them from entering and infecting cells. It is the accumulation of immune cells and dead germs that causes lymph nodes to become hard, swollen, and tender when the body is fighting a disease. You

LINK TO

may have experienced swollen lymph nodes in the neck when suffering a throat infection. This shows that the body's defense systems are activated.

If the lymphatic system is sluggish, then toxins are able to accumulate and circulate around the body, excess fluid builds up, and the body's defense is compromised. This can lead to many different symptoms, including fatigue, nasal and sinus congestion, susceptibility to coughs and colds, frequent headaches, puffiness, disturbed sleep, and dull skin and hair.

THE LYMPHATICS: BENEFITS OF SELF-MASSAGE

Self-massage has many beneficial effects on the lymphatic system.

◆ A more efficient flow of lymph through the intestine ensures that all body tissues are well supplied with the fats they need.

◆ Speedy removal of metabolic wastes, toxins, and excess fluid helps the body's tissues function more efficiently.

◆ Vital proteins are collected from the cells and returned to the blood for distribution to other areas.

◆ The body's defense systems are aided in their fight against infections and in providing immunity to future disease.

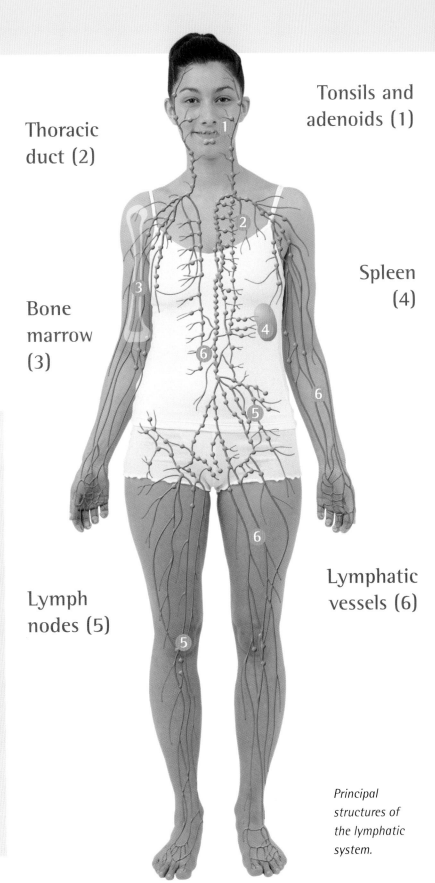

Thoracic duct (2)

Tonsils and adenoids (1)

Spleen (4)

Bone marrow (3)

Lymph nodes (5)

Lymphatic vessels (6)

Principal structures of the lymphatic system.

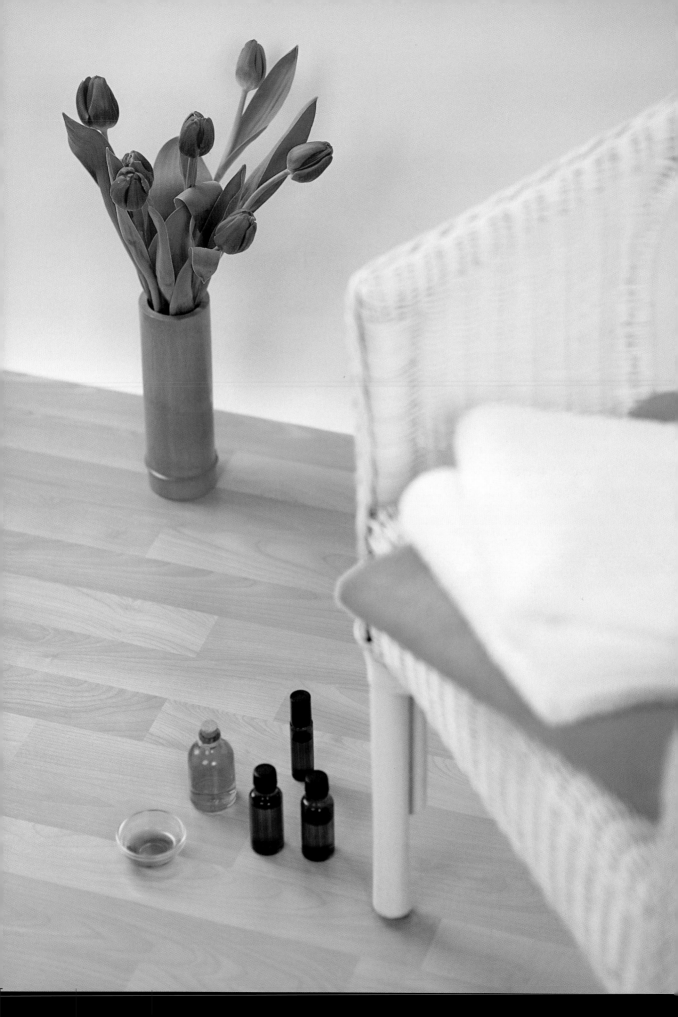

2 GETTING PREPARED

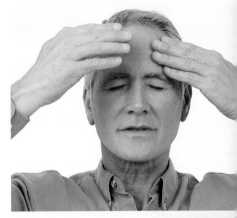

Sometimes you need instant relief from aches and pains. When a headache strikes or a cramp seizes your foot, there is little time for preparation. You want to ease the problem as quickly as possible. However, there are occasions when a little forward planning can boost the positive effects of self-massage.

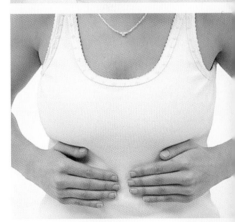

◆ Set time aside to complete your massage sequence—even if it is only five minutes. Early evening is best for a relaxing massage, for example, especially if you have time afterward to sit quietly and enjoy a sense of peace and tranquillity.

◆ Some of the sequences are best performed in privacy. Try to find a quiet corner in the office or find a few moments when you know you will not be disturbed.

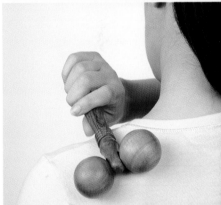

◆ If possible, remove your watch or any large rings and bracelets, as these could get in the way and may scratch your skin. You may prefer to remove your shoes, too, as this adds to the relaxation factor.

◆ Check your posture so you can massage yourself without straining or overstretching. Twisting your body into awkward positions will only add to your aches and pains. Use props such as small pillows or a towel to support your neck and knees when lying on the floor, and if there is no carpet, protect your back with an exercise mat or folded blanket.

◆ Massage oils are greasy and can easily stain. If using them, protect clothes and furniture with towels or paper towels.

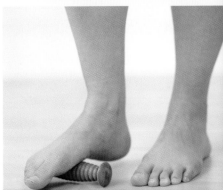

Safety first

The massage movements described in this book have been chosen because, if followed correctly, they are safe to use on yourself without any formal training. However, it is important not to launch straight into a massage sequence without your doctor's advice. These basic guidelines will help ensure optimum effectiveness and safety for your self-massage.

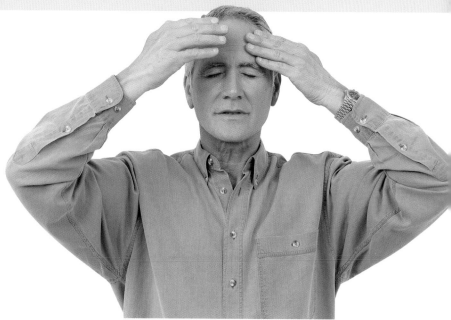

Follow these simple suggestions to help prolong the benefits of self-massage:

◆ Drink plenty of water and herbal teas to speed up the elimination of toxins from your body. Cut back on tea, alcohol, coffee, and colas, which act like a diuretic, increasing the flow of urine from the body.

◆ Avoid eating heavy meals right after self-massage. The demands of digestion will divert energy away from the natural healing process. Light snacks and fresh fruit are best.

◆ Occasionally, people have a mild reaction to massage. This may lead to a slight headache, increased perspiration, or increased urination. These reactions usually pass within 24 hours and should be considered a positive sign that the body is rebalancing and cleansing itself.

◆ Remember, massage should never be painful. Nor should it be irritating or cause dizziness. So stop if any movement feels uncomfortable or unpleasant; we all find certain movements more or less beneficial and enjoyable than other ones. Experiment to find the level of pressure that feels best for you. After all, one of the advantages of self-massage is that you can adapt your method so that it exactly suits your needs.

◆ It may be tempting to enhance the relaxing effects of massage with a drink, but it is impossible to know how you will react to massage under the influence of alcohol or other stimulants, so do not take the risk. For more safety advice, see box (right).

HEALTH CHECK

There may be a few occasions when it is not appropriate to give yourself a massage or when you need to take extra care. So check for the following:

◆ ONGOING MEDICAL CONDITIONS: It is wise to seek advice from your medical practitioner if you have a chronic medical condition such as a serious heart disorder, epilepsy, diabetes, and/or you are taking strong medication.

◆ RECENT INJURY: Avoid areas where there has been recent injury, including sprains, strains, fractures, and whiplash. Massage could be painful and make the injury worse. Wait until you are sure the injury has healed.

◆ THROMBOSIS: If you have a history of thrombosis or embolism, be very cautious when massaging the limbs and use only light strokes—or avoid the area altogether. There is a slight risk that deep massage may encourage a clot or fragment to break away and enter the bloodstream.

◆ PREGNANCY: In pregnancy, use only gentle massage, especially during the first three months. Be especially careful

with abdominal massage, using only caressing strokes as suggested in "Pregnancy" (pages 78–81).

◆ INFECTIOUS SKIN CONDITIONS: Avoid massaging over areas of skin or scalp that show signs of infection or contagious disease, as massage may irritate and/or spread the disorder.

◆ RECENT SURGERY: Do not massage over new scar tissue or an area that recently underwent surgery, as it may hinder the healing process.

◆ VARICOSE VEINS: Treat protruding or varicose veins with care. Brush lightly over them without exerting any pressure.

◆ MIGRAINE ATTACK: Massage during a migraine attack could make the symptoms worse.

◆ ARTHRITIC JOINTS: Avoid deep massage over arthritic, swollen, inflamed, or painful joints. Deep massage might offer short-term relief, but it generates heat that can aggravate the condition in the long term. Light, gentle strokes are more beneficial.

◆ FRAGILE BONES: Avoid strong pressure on fragile bones, as deep massage could cause a fracture.

◆ LUMPS, BUMPS, AND BITES: Avoid massaging directly over warts, moles, skin tags, bruises, cuts, bites, areas of sunburn, and lumps and bumps.

◆ SWOLLEN LYMPH NODES: Never massage over swollen lymph nodes, as this may interfere with the body's natural defense mechanisms.

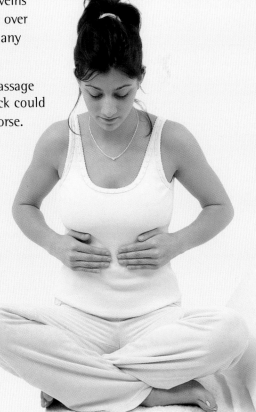

Self-massage made easier

When you want to massage those tricky areas that are out of reach, a self-massage tool can be a wonderful asset. Here is a selection of some of the tools available to help you knead, roll, and brush away your aches and pains.

Foot rollers

Remove your shoes and sit in a chair. Place your foot on the roller and roll it forward and backward under your sole to help create comforting warmth and to ease stiffness.

Body massagers

Hold the handle firmly with one hand and gently roll the balls all over your body. These are great for targeting tension and fatigue in legs, arms, and shoulders. Massagers can be used over light clothing or directly on bare skin, or when using a massage oil either on its own or mixed with essential oils (see pages 32–35).

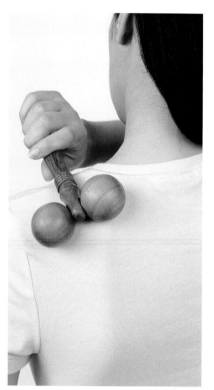

Stress balls

To strengthen and mobilize your hands (and alleviate stress), use a small soft rubber ball. Squeeze, roll, and mold it slowly in your hands so that you exercise your muscles without overdoing it. Keep one in your desk drawer to help you keep calm during times of increased stress.

Chinese hand balls

These small balls, available from specialty shops, work by stimulating the acupressure points on the hands and increasing the flow of vital energy through the body. Hold two balls in the palm of one hand and circle them

When under pressure at work, body massagers can help ease away the tension that builds up in the muscles of the back, shoulders, arms, and thighs.

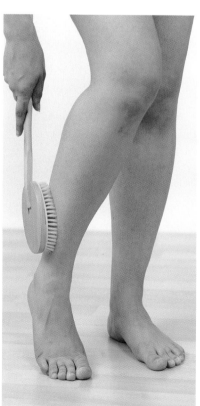

around each other in your palm and fingers. The more you practice, the easier it becomes. You can choose balls with a musical accompaniment to add to the enjoyment.

Dry skin brushes

Set aside a couple of minutes each morning for body brushing, using a loofah or firm-bristled brush directly on your skin. Do not wet the brush or use any oil or body moisturizer. Dry skin brushing helps boost blood and lymph circulation, sloughs off dull, dead cells on the skin surface, and stimulates production of sebum, the skin's natural moisturizer.

1. Start at your feet and brush up your legs with long, firm strokes.
2. Move up to your thighs and buttocks, arms and shoulders, always directing the strokes toward the heart.
3. Use gentle pressure on your abdomen, always working in a circular clockwise direction.
4. Brush lightly on your breasts, but avoid the delicate nipples.
5. Finish with an energizing shower to set you up for the day ahead.

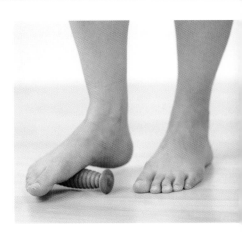

A foot roller offers a great way to ease tension and stiffness in the feet after a tiring day spent at work or at the mall.

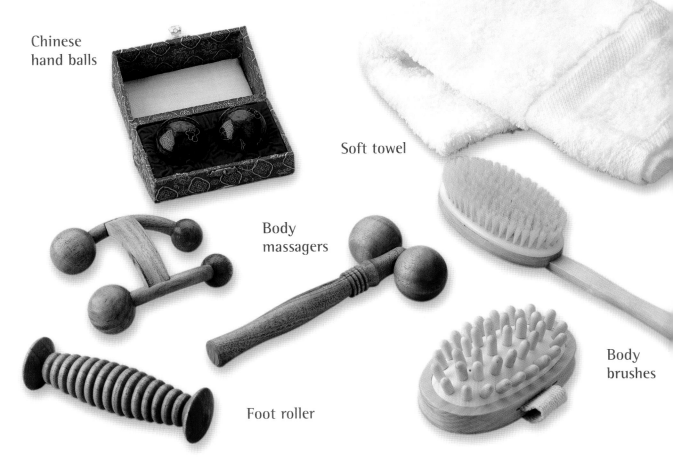

Chinese hand balls

Soft towel

Body massagers

Foot roller

Body brushes

Oils for self-massage

The tradition of using natural vegetable oils and aromatic essential oils as a valuable adjunct to massage goes back centuries. The self-massage techniques described in this book can easily be performed through clothes without the need for oils. However, there may be occasions when the use of oils can complement your self-massage.

Before choosing and using oils for therapeutic purposes, it is important to distinguish between the types of massage oils and their uses. There are two main types of massage oil—carrier oils and pure essential oils.

Carrier oils, or base oils, as they are often called, dilute essential oils to make them safe to use and act as a lubricant to make the massage more flowing. Natural vegetable oils are rich in vitamins, proteins, and minerals to help moisturize, nourish, and strengthen skin and hair.

Pure essential oils are concentrated plant extracts. A few drops only are mixed with carrier oils to provide extra beneficial effects—a form of treatment called aromatherapy. Pure essential oils are featured on pages 34-35. The following are the top carrier oils used in self-massage.

Sweet almond

This popular oil is light and smooth to use. Sweet almond oil helps to protect and nourish the skin and is especially beneficial for dry, sensitive, and irritated skin conditions.
CAUTION: Not to be confused with bitter almond, which can be toxic. Sweet almond oil is generally well tolerated, but do not use if you have a nut allergy. Use another carrier oil instead.

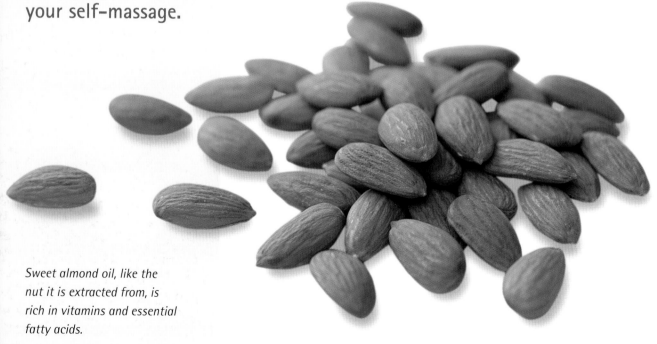

Sweet almond oil, like the nut it is extracted from, is rich in vitamins and essential fatty acids.

Jojoba

Jojoba (pronounced ho-HO-ba) oil, a liquid wax that is often used in massage, has a similar chemical structure to sebum, the skin's natural cleanser and moisturizer, and is beneficial for all skin types. It contains vitamin E, a natural antioxidant, and thus has antiaging properties. Generally well tolerated.
CAUTION: Although jojoba oil is wonderfully nourishing, it is fairly expensive, so you may prefer to dilute it with another carrier oil, such as sweet almond or sunflower oil.

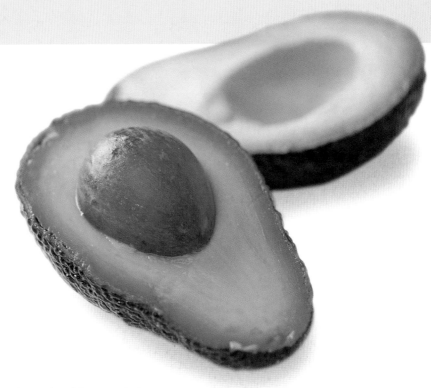

Avocado oil is extracted from dried slices of the fleshy portion of the avocado fruit. Look for unrefined, cold-pressed oil for the best quality.

Avocado

This nutritious oil is deep green in color with a distinctive aroma. It acts as a wonderful emollient, softening and smoothing the skin. Avocado oil has antiwrinkle properties and is often favored by people with dry, mature skins.
CAUTION: Avocado oil is fairly thick, so you may prefer to mix it with a lighter carrier oil.

Evening primrose

This oil is rich in essential fatty acids, especially gamma linoleic acid (GLA), which is often used to treat premenstrual syndrome and other menstrual problems and menopausal symptoms. Evening primrose oil is also a good skin softener and is particularly useful for dry, aging, or chapped skins.

CAUTION: Generally well tolerated. Evening primrose oil can become sticky during massage, so it is best added to a lighter carrier oil such as sunflower oil.

Sunflower

Organic sunflower oil is becoming increasingly popular in aromatherapy and massage, because it is safe for people of all ages and skin types. It is nutritious and moisturizing and mixes well with other carrier oils and pure essential oils.

CAUTION: For aromatherapy and massage, choose oil extracted from organically grown plants to ensure purity and safety.

◆ Carrier oils can be used on their own or blended with pure essential oils for massage or in baths. The following pages offer suggestions for blending and using pure essential oils.

Pure essential oils

Essential oils are nongreasy and highly concentrated essences extracted from aromatic plants. Only tiny quantities are needed to have a powerful impact on mind, body, and emotions. Their distinctive aromas have a profound influence on moods—certain scents can relax and soothe or invigorate and uplift.

The therapeutic ingredients of pure essential oils are inhaled and/or absorbed through the skin and into the bloodstream, where they travel around the body to fulfill their healing functions. This is the basis of aromatherapy.

The following are the most popular oils used in massage. They are safe for home use as directed. To find out about other essential oils, ask a fully qualified aromatherapist for advice.

Lavender

This is such a versatile oil that it may be the only one you need. A natural sedative, lavender induces calm and promotes restful sleep. It also has painkilling properties, so it is useful for easing headaches and alleviating muscular aches and pains. It also helps boost the immune system. Well tolerated.

Geranium

Geranium has a balancing effect on mind and body. It aids the circulation and stimulates lymph drainage. Geranium oil can calm an overactive mind and is a useful tonic for low moods and mild depression especially associated with premenstrual syndrome and menopause.
CAUTION: Test before using, as it may irritate sensitive skin.

Frankincense

Frankincense is a highly aromatic oil that can induce deep, slow breathing, so it is often used during meditation to promote concentrated and focused thought. Frankincense is a natural rejuvenator and can be added to carrier oils to help moisturize and soothe dry and mature skin. Well tolerated.

SAFE USE OF ESSENTIAL OILS

◆ Avoid using pure essential oils during pregnancy, when breastfeeding, or on babies and children unless advised by a fully qualified aromatherapist.

◆ Check safety warnings on oils before use, and avoid if likely to cause irritation or aggravate a medical condition.

◆ Never apply essential oils undiluted (except lavender). For massage, always dilute with a carrier oil in correct proportions.

◆ Do not take internally. If oils are consumed accidentally, get immediate medical help. If oil gets into the eyes, rinse with sweet almond oil to ease the stinging. If in doubt, seek medical assistance.

◆ Store in a cool, dark place away from children and pets.

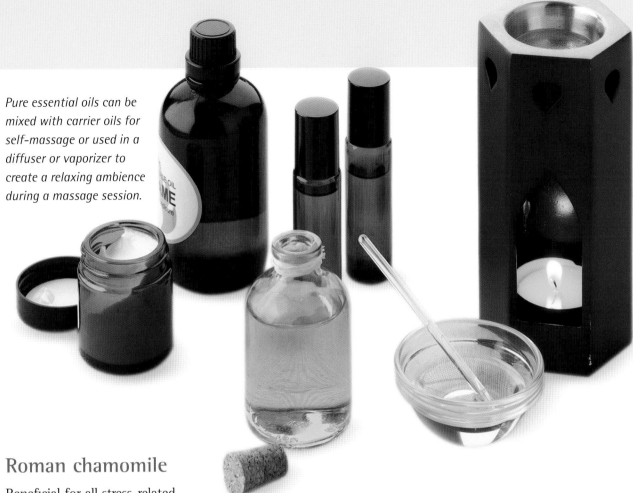

Pure essential oils can be mixed with carrier oils for self-massage or used in a diffuser or vaporizer to create a relaxing ambience during a massage session.

Roman chamomile

Beneficial for all stress-related conditions, chamomile has a soothing effect on mind and body. It relieves muscular pains and cramps, and can ease the tension and anxiety associated with premenstrual syndrome and menopause.
CAUTION: Test before using, as it may irritate sensitive skin.

Rosemary

This is an invigorating, energizing oil that lifts mental fatigue and lethargy and refreshes and clears the mind. It improves and aids memory and can ease headaches. Rosemary also stimulates blood circulation and warms the body.

CAUTION: Do not use if you have high blood pressure or epilepsy. Because it is a stimulating oil, it should be avoided before bedtime.

Eucalyptus

A stimulating and warming oil, eucalyptus is particularly useful in steam inhalations to help ease respiratory problems and clear congestion. It can also help strengthen the immune system to fight infection.
CAUTION: Use in low dilutions and test before using, as it can irritate the skin. Seek professional advice

if taking homeopathic remedies, because eucalyptus may counteract the benefits of the treatment.

WARNING

If you have sensitive skin, do a patch test before massaging. Mix 1 drop of your chosen oil in a teaspoon of carrier oil and rub a little behind your ears or on your wrist. Leave for 24 hours. If you notice any redness or itchiness, do not use the oil. Rinse off with cold water.

Aromatherapy for health

Carrier oils and pure essential oils can be used in a wide variety of ways to help alleviate many everyday ailments.

Carrier oils also have therapeutic effects, so they can be used on their own—to moisturize and nourish the skin, for example—or combined with pure essential oils. When blending oil for massage, always use a safe amount of essential oil. The recommended dose for home use is 1 to 2 drops of a single pure essential oil to every 1 teaspoon (5 ml) of carrier oil. Do not be tempted to add more. Essential oils are highly concentrated and powerful substances.

Begin by measuring the carrier oil and pouring it into a small bowl, bottle, or container. With practice, you will discover how much carrier oil you need for self-massage, but as a general guideline, use 1 teaspoon (5 ml) for face massage and 3 teaspoons (15 ml) for a full-body massage. Add the correct number of drops of pure essential oil. Stir with a clean spoon or cocktail stick.

Oil is best applied warm to encourage the absorption of the natural-healing chemicals. Wash your hands, then warm them by rubbing together or immersing in a bowl of warm water for a few minutes. Place some oil in the palms of your hands and rub together until well covered and warm to touch. Add more oil as necessary during the massage.

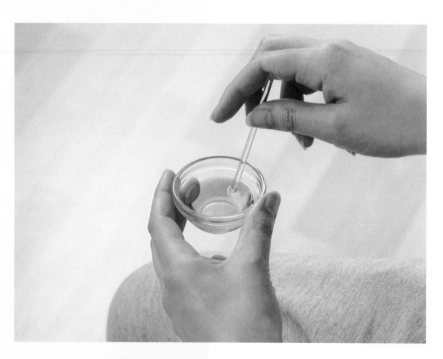

Baths

One of the easiest ways of using oils is to add them to a bath. You can use carrier oils on their own,

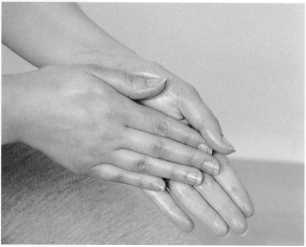

If using oil for self-massage, make sure you prepare enough to cover the area of skin you are massaging, and rub your hands together to warm the oil before applying to the skin.

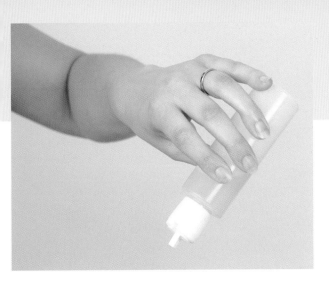

a tissue and inhale when required. To store the aroma, wrap the tissue in foil until needed. Inhale deeply 2–3 times as required. CAUTION: **Steam inhalation is not recommended for asthmatics.**

but for a wonderfully therapeutic bath, combine 1 teaspoon (5 ml) of carrier oil with up to 5 drops of your chosen pure essential oil. Now fill the bath with water. Add the mixture to your bath and gently agitate the water. Close the windows so that you get maximum benefit from the aromatic atmosphere.

Keep the water temperature warm or cool. If the water is too hot, the oils will evaporate too quickly. A warm bath is more relaxing, and a cool bath is invigorating and stimulating.

You can add essential oils directly to the water, but since they do not dissolve, they will either float or sink. To avoid a greasy ring around the bath or bowl, add essential oils to an emulsifier such as whole milk or fragrance-free bath lotion instead of carrier oil.

To soak hands or feet, fill a large bowl with warm or cool water and add carrier oil on its own or blend with essential oils.

Inhalation

This traditional method of inhaling aromatic vapors is still one of the most effective for clearing the respiratory tract and relieving catarrh and sinus problems. Eucalyptus oil is widely used for steam inhalations. Boil around 4 cups (950 ml) of water and pour into a bowl. Put 2 drops of oil directly onto the water. Put a towel or cloth over your head. Close your eyes and lean over the bowl, not too close to the water. Inhale the aromatic steam for up to 10 minutes or as long as is comfortable. Repeat several times a day as necessary. Alternatively, place 1 or 2 drops (no more) of neat essential oil on

Compresses

Compresses can be hot or cold. A hot compress is good for cramps, chest congestion, and muscular pains. A cold compress is best for eye strain, headaches, hangovers, or inflammation. Fill a bowl with $3\frac{1}{2}$ fl. oz. (100 ml) of hot or cold water. Add 1 drop of your chosen essential oil. Now lay a piece of flannel or clean cotton on the surface of the water to absorb the oil. Squeeze out any excess water and place the compress over the affected area. Leave in place for up to 2 hours. Reapply as often as you wish.

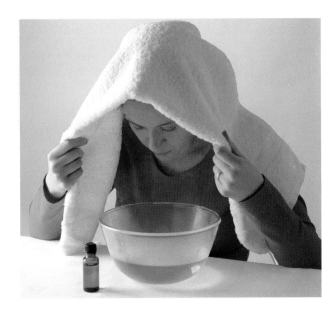

Steam inhalation is a good way to relieve chest and sinus conditions and also relieve some skin disorders.

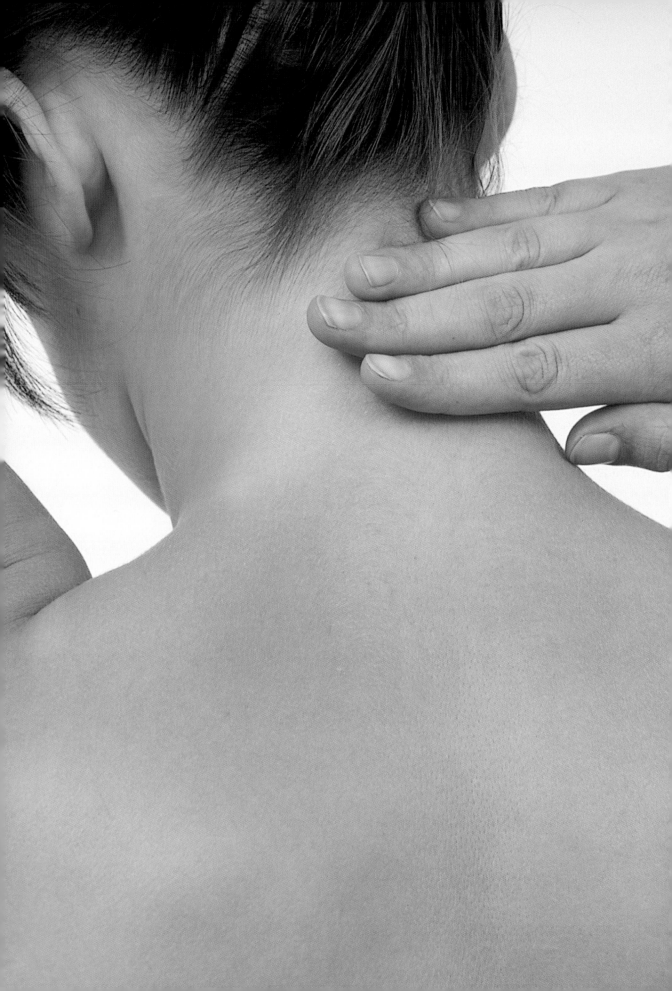

3 BASIC MASSAGE TECHNIQUES

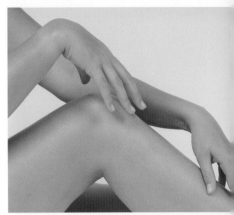

The step-by-step sequences in this book are based on 10 simple, safe, and effective techniques that have an effect on the mind and body as a whole. You will soon master these techniques and gain an intuitive understanding of when to use them. One of the joys of self-massage is that you know what feels right for you. If you are using these moves on another person, be careful not to press too hard or it could be painful. Conversely, pressing too lightly can be irritating or ticklish.

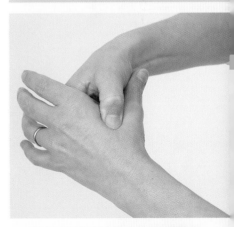

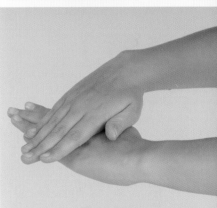

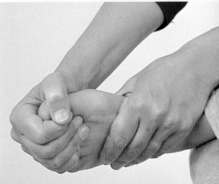

Holding

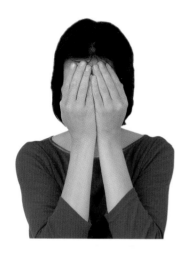

Cupping the palms of your hands over your eyes and holding for a minute offer a safe darkness that helps refresh tired eyes.

Simple holds can be surprisingly calming, and their effectiveness should never be underestimated, even in self-massage. While we usually associate massage with movement, holding can bring a welcome stillness that can be most comforting at times of stress or tension. Think how we instinctively reach out to hold someone's hand or give a quiet hug in a crisis. The holding technique allows us to offer the same reassurance to ourselves when we need it.

When holding, try the following:
- Use the whole surface of your palms and fingers to gain optimum contact.
- Maintain the hold for at least half a minute, longer if possible.
- Experiment by adding a little pressure; it gives a different feel to a technique.
- For a reinforced hold, place one hand on top of the other.
- Close your eyes and take some deep breaths to encourage further relaxation.
- To switch off from circling thoughts, think of a color or concentrate on the steady ebb and flow of your breathing.
- Release your hold very gradually so that your hands gently draw away.

To add variation to a hold, try gently rocking the area at the same time. Keep the movement slow, reassuring, and rhythmic.

Where to use
It is safe to use the holding technique on any part of your body that can be comfortably accessed with the palms of one or both hands. Holding is particularly calming on head, face, abdomen, and feet.

Benefits
Holding brings a sense of stillness that can be so difficult to obtain in our busy world. It gives you time to stop, focus, and refresh your mind. The heat generated by the palms of your hands adds to the relaxing effect. For extra benefit, rub your hands together before applying the hold.

Holding your hands on your head for a minute can be so soothing that it may be all that is needed to lift a mild tension headache.

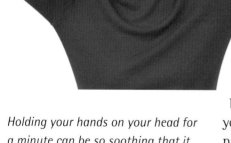

Holding your feet provides warmth and comfort and is especially beneficial after a tiring day.

Feathering

As the name suggests, this is the lightest and softest of all the massage strokes, and it feels wonderfully soothing, especially at the start or end of a massage.

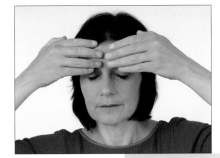

Light, featherlike strokes on the forehead can soothe a furrowed brow and release tension.

When applying this technique, try the following:

• Imagine that you are gently stroking your skin with a feather.

• Relax your hands and let the pads of your fingers stroke the skin in a long, sweeping motion in all directions over the body.

• Ensure that your fingertips barely touch the surface of your skin, and avoid contact with the palms of your hands.

• Release your touch very, very slowly at the end of each stroke so that your hands float away smoothly.

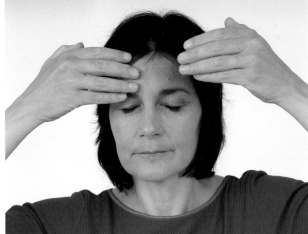

Your hands can work together or alternately so that each stroke follows immediately after the previous one in a wavelike motion. Much of the pleasure of the technique lies in the repetition, which gently calms your sensory nerve endings, so continue feathering for as long as it feels good.

Where to use

The feathering technique is suitable for all parts of the body and can be used at any time during the massage. It is such a safe stroke that it is often performed on children and frail people and is ideal for use in pregnancy. Feathering feels especially soothing on the forehead and face. It is best avoided on ticklish areas of the body.

Benefits

Feathering can be used at any time to relax the sensory nerve endings and to induce feelings of calm and peace. Feathering brings a sense of lightness to mind and body that can help to ease anxiety, combat stress, and promote a good night's sleep.

Feathering along the tops of the hands and arms brings a sense of relaxation to the whole body.

Light stroking

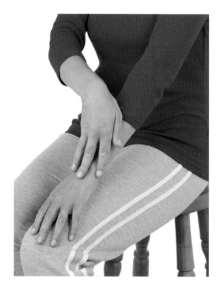

Gentle stroking on the tops of the hands and wrists has an instant calming effect. Try this simple technique when you need to stay cool and composed as tensions rise at work.

Light stroking is one of the most versatile of all the massage techniques and can be performed with the palms of your hands, your fingers or thumbs, and can follow any direction. It is the kind of smooth, rhythmical stroking action we naturally use when reassuring a loved one or nurturing a pet.

When applying this technique, try the following:
• Keep your hands and fingers supple and slightly cupped so they naturally mold to the bends and curves of the part being massaged.
• Use a light pressure so that your hands or fingers glide over the surface of the skin.

Light stroking can be performed in straight sweeps or in a comforting, circular movement over a small or large area of the body. You can stroke with one hand or both hands together. You can also use alternate hands, one following the other, in a flowing rhythm.

Where to use
Light stroking can be safely applied to all areas of the body. It is a relaxing technique to use during times of stress. It also helps to warm and prepare the body for deeper massage and to soothe an area following more stimulating massage techniques.

Benefits
Slow, flowing stroking helps soothe sensory nerve endings and promotes a sense of relaxation throughout the whole body. It has an almost soporific effect on mind and body, easing mental stress and helping you unwind after a busy day.

Raking
A variation on stroking is a technique known as raking. Make your hands into a clawlike shape and use the pads of your stiff fingers to stroke in long, sweeping movements. Keep your fingers rigid and apply a firm, but not too deep, pressure. You can rake with both hands together or alternate one hand after the other.

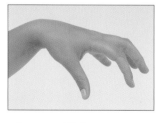

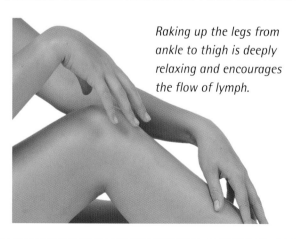

Raking up the legs from ankle to thigh is deeply relaxing and encourages the flow of lymph.

Deep stroking

This technique, which is sometimes called effleurage, is similar to light stroking but is a firmer, smoothing action in the direction of the heart. It follows naturally from light stroking in a massage sequence. Deep stroking is usually performed with the palms of both hands. The strokes are long and flowing. The hands glide lightly over your skin, following the natural curves of your body. When using this stroke, your hands generally cover as large an area of skin as possible. On smaller areas, however, you can use one hand, the soft pads of the thumbs, or your fingers.

When applying this technique, try the following:
• Let your hands run smoothly over the skin, molding to the contours of your body. Keep the wrists flexible and the hands supple and flowing in a long, continuous sequence.
• When working on the arms or legs, deep strokes always follow the direction of the venous flow back to the heart or toward the nearest set of lymph nodes.
• Make your pressure firmer on the upward stroke toward the heart, using a lighter touch on the return movement.

Where to use
Deep stroking is safe to use on all parts of the body. It is often used to link massage movements together so that the massage flows more effectively. Deep stroking is used after deeper massage techniques to aid the flow of excess blood to the heart or lymph or the nearest set of lymph nodes (see pages 24–25).

Stroking in a circular clockwise direction on the abdomen can help calm the stomach and relieve digestive disorders.

Benefits
Deep stroking soothes sensory nerve endings, inducing general physical and psychological relaxation. Firm strokes help boost blood and lymph circulation, and warm the area in preparation for deeper massage. The increased warmth soothes tired and aching muscles.

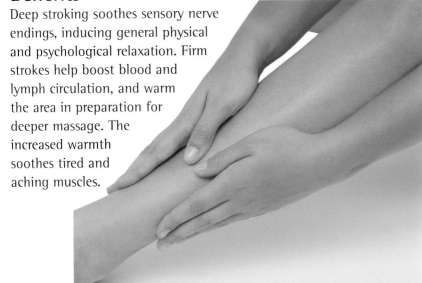

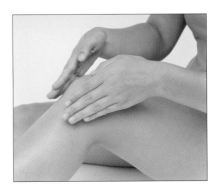

Use the deep-stroking technique from your ankles to thighs to boost poor circulation and gently ease everyday aches and pains.

Kneading

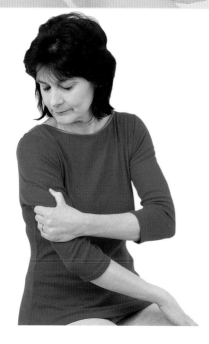

This movement, as you might imagine, is rather like kneading dough. It is a deeper movement than stroking and is generally used on fleshy areas only. The technique involves gently lifting an area of muscle mass, then compressing, rolling, or squeezing it before releasing.

Kneading can be performed with a light or deep pressure depending on the area you are massaging. Keep the pressure fairly gentle on smaller areas of flesh and the more superficial muscles, such as those on the face, but use a much firmer pressure on larger, thicker muscles, such as those in the thighs. On larger areas within easy reach, such as your buttocks, you can use both hands alternately to knead the soft tissues. On other areas of your body, it may be more appropriate to use one hand only.

When applying this technique, try the following:
- Begin by placing your hands on the muscle, then gently mold your fingers around the flesh and roll it between your fingers and the heels of your hands.
- Over smaller areas, such as the hands and feet, knead the flesh between fingers and thumbs.
- Keep your hands relaxed and supple using a slow, rhythmic movement.

Kneading your upper arm with one hand relaxes taut muscles and helps boost the circulation of blood and lymph in the arms.

Finger or thumb rotations

A useful kneading technique is finger or thumb rotations. The fleshy pads of the fingers or thumbs work on small areas in a circular motion, increasing pressure on the upward half of the circle, decreasing pressure on the downward half. Once you complete the circle, glide the hand to the next area in a slow, flowing movement, without losing contact or rhythm, to start another rotation. Apply pressure as deep as you can tolerate (but it should not be painful). Avoid pinching or working too long in one area, as this can cause pain.

Small, circular kneading rotations with fingers and thumbs around the ankle can help refresh and relax stiff, tired, and puffy ankles.

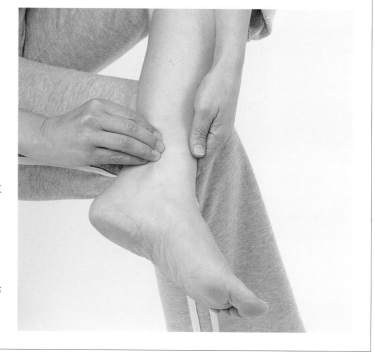

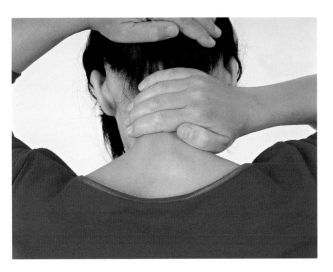

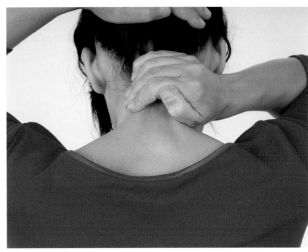

• Use a deep but comfortable pressure. Your hands do not glide over the surface of the skin but press much deeper, so you can feel the underlying tissues moving and detect any nodules of tension. As you work, you will feel these areas steadily relaxing beneath your touch, leaving you feeling more relaxed.

Larger kneading movements using the palms of your hands can relieve tension in the muscles along the tops of your shoulders and upper back.

Where to use

Kneading can be used on all areas of muscle mass that can be reached by the hands, or fingers and thumbs. It is often used to boost blood and lymph circulation in the thighs or to relax muscles in the shoulders and upper back. Gentle kneading between fingers and thumbs is useful for taut muscles in the hands and feet. However, kneading tends to create heat, so do not use it over arthritic, painful, hot, or inflamed joints.

Benefits

Kneading can be very effective in reducing pain, tension, and stiffness in overworked muscles. It also stimulates blood and lymph flow. The rhythmic compression and relaxation of your hands act like a pump to boost the flow of blood back to the heart and to push lymph to the nearest set of lymph nodes to be cleansed and filtered. This cleansing action is enhanced if kneading is followed by deep stroking in the direction of the heart or lymph nodes. Kneading also stimulates the sebaceous glands to secrete sebum, the body's natural moisturizer, which keeps skin smooth and gives hair a glossy sheen.

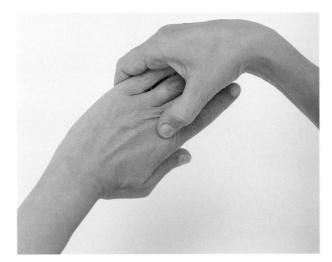

Gentle thumb kneading along the grooves on the top of the hand can help refresh tired hands.

Pressures

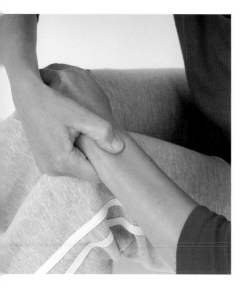

Pressures are fairly deep and precise movements applied to localized areas of muscle tension. They are valuable in self-massage because they are effective without oils and are easily performed through clothes. Pressures are usually applied with the pads of fingers or thumbs, but you can use the heel of the hand, knuckles, or even elbow if your hands get tired. Fingers do not glide over the skin, as in stroking or kneading. Pressure is applied; then the fingers or thumbs are lifted before moving on to the next spot. Massage tools (see pages 30-31) are a useful way of performing pressures without straining fingers and thumbs. There are two main types of pressures: static and circular.

When applying this technique, try the following:
For static pressures:
• Hold the pressure on a single point for a count of 3 to 5; then very slowly release and move to the next area.
• To help reinforce the pressure, place your second finger on top of your first finger when applying pressures.
• Inhale as you exert pressure, and exhale as you release pressure.
• Static pressures should not be confused with acupressure. This involves applying pressure to acupoints, which are specific sites located along energy pathways (known as meridians) in the body (see page 51).

Applying static pressures on the lower arm helps release the tension that can build up after spending long hours working at a computer.

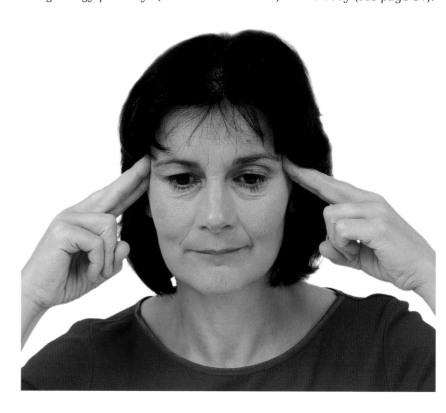

Circular pressures on the temples help relieve tension in an area where taut muscles are a common cause of headaches and eyestrain.

For circular pressures:
• Move the skin against the underlying tissue in a circular motion, gradually increasing the pressure as you work deeper into the area. After a few seconds very slowly release; then move to the next area.
• Vary the size and depth of circles.
• Do not confuse circular pressures with finger or thumb rotations, where a mass of muscle is massaged—with the pressure increasing on the upward half of the circle and decreasing on the downward half. Pressures are more specific moves, with a gradual increase in intensity.

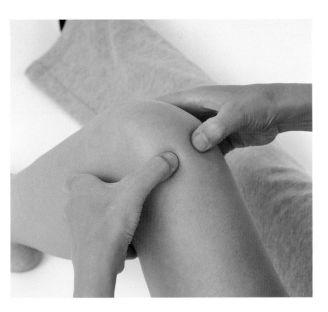
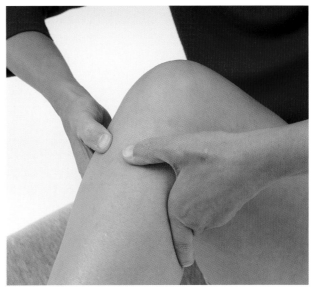

Where to use
Pressures can be applied to most parts of the body, especially muscles and around joints, but avoid using on sensitive or delicate areas, such as the abdomen. If applying deep pressures, always warm the area first, using light, superficial strokes, and follow with gentle stroking.

Static pressures around the knee joint can help release any tightness and increase mobility.

Benefits
Deep pressures are especially beneficial in targeting areas of tightness or adhesions in muscle fibers, such as those along the upper shoulders. Pressures are also used around joints to loosen any adhesions and aid mobility. Lighter pressures are used on the face to feel for taut muscles and help disperse any tension. Pressures help boost blood and lymph circulation in the local area, promoting healing by increasing supplies of oxygen and nutrients and ensuring more efficient removal of excess fluid and waste products.

Beating

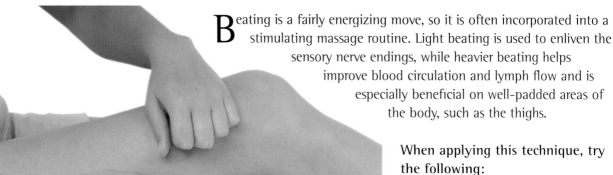

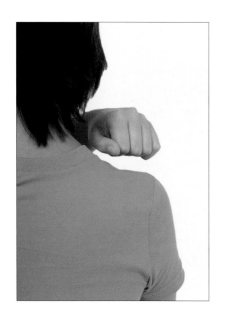

Beating is a fairly energizing move, so it is often incorporated into a stimulating massage routine. Light beating is used to enliven the sensory nerve endings, while heavier beating helps improve blood circulation and lymph flow and is especially beneficial on well-padded areas of the body, such as the thighs.

Beating the large muscles in your buttocks and thighs can help break up fatty deposits and soften areas of fatty tissue, improving skin texture.

When applying this technique, try the following:

- Make your hands into loose fists with your fingers really relaxed. Keep the wrists flexible.
- Use the sides of your fists or the backs of loosely clenched fingers and the heels of the hands.
- Strike the flesh with a springy, drumming movement, using both hands alternately in a rhythm. Your hands bounce back as soon as they land on the skin. The pressure can be light or slightly heavier, depending on the area being massaged.
- On smaller areas, beat with one hand only.
- Begin with a soft, slow strike, and gradually build up to a more rapid, forceful action.
- Move up and down or across the area so that you don't work over the same spot for too long.

Where to use

Heavier beating is usually performed over fleshy areas, such as the thighs and buttocks, or the dense muscle across the top of the shoulders. Be careful not to strike any bony prominences, as this can be painful. Prepare the area by stroking, and finish with gentle strokes to soothe sensory nerve endings. *Warning: Never use a beating technique over the kidneys or spine.*

Benefits

Beating helps stimulate blood circulation and warms the area, leaving a tingling sensation in the muscles. It can be a very effective way to soften areas of hard, fatty tissue and may help tone slack muscles. Fast beating produces an invigorating sensation and is generally very refreshing and uplifting; a slower speed is more relaxing.

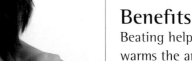

Beating along the fleshy area on the tops of the shoulders boosts the circulation to the muscles.

Rubbing

A n invigorating, warming movement, rubbing the skin is our natural response when we feel chilly—and a useful technique for self-massage. You can use the palm, heel, or side of your hands for rubbing, depending on the size of the area. Alternatively, you can rub using the pads of two or more fingers.

When applying this technique, try the following:
• Hold your fingers straight and keep your wrists flexible.
• Use a brisk sawing action with hands or fingers, working backward and forward over the surface of the skin in any direction.
• Ensure that your hand or fingers move swiftly over the area. Do not stay in the same place for too long.

An adaptation of the move is to hold your hands in loosely clenched fists and apply the same rubbing technique with the backs of your fingers and the heel of your hands.

Rubbing up the back of the neck with the flats of your fingers helps ease stiffness in this tension hot spot.

Where to use
Rubbing can be applied to all parts of the body, although only a very gentle pressure should be applied on sensitive areas, such as the face. It is particularly effective on the scalp, shoulders, and neck.

Benefits
As you would imagine, rubbing stimulates local blood circulation and generates heat in the area. Rubbing helps relax and loosen tense muscles while producing an invigorating effect on mind and body.

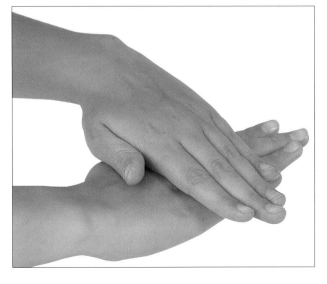

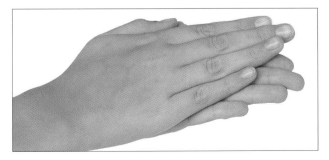

Rubbing the hands before massage is a good way to warm and relax the palms and fingers.

Tapping

This technique involves striking the skin, then releasing in a rapid, rhythmical way, like using a percussion instrument. It is a brisk, energizing movement. You can use your fingertips or the palms or backs of your hands, depending on the area being massaged. Sometimes you might choose to tap with one hand, or you may prefer to use both hands, tapping simultaneously or alternately. It is a good idea to try different variations until you find the one that suits you best.

Tone the muscles under the chin by lightly tapping with the backs of your fingers.

When applying this technique, try the following:
- Keep your wrists flexible, and use your hands or fingers to tap the skin with a light, springy movement. Your hands or fingers bounce back up as soon as they land on the skin.
- Allow your hands to move around rapidly to cover the whole area with the tapping.
- It is best to start slowly and lightly, and gradually make the move faster and more invigorating to avoid an abrupt shock.
- If you are using your fingertips, then it helps to imagine you are playing the piano or drumming your fingers impatiently on a table.
- Tap quickly, energetically, and firmly without being too heavy-handed. It is a rhythmical move, but there is no need for your fingers to tap in any particular order.

Where to use

Tapping is safe on all parts of the body. Gentle tapping is often used on delicate, sensitive areas, such as the face. Before using deep tapping, always warm and prepare the area with stroking movements.

Benefits

Light tapping is soothing and relaxing for tension-related conditions, such as jaw ache or eyestrain. Slightly deeper tapping stimulates blood and lymph flow and can be part of an energizing, circulation-enhancing routine. Tapping also tones muscles and stimulates the nerves, awakening mind and body. Use to improve your concentration and boost energy.

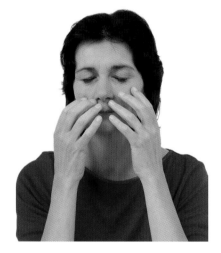

Tapping with your fingertips on your face has a stimulating and refreshing effect.

Tapping one hand with the flats of the fingers of your free hand can create warmth and aid blood and lymph flow.

Acupressure

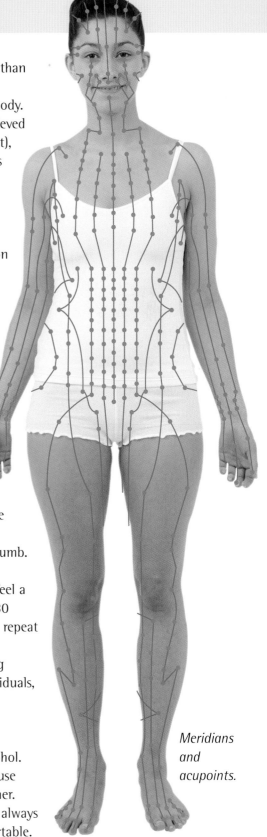

Acupressure is a branch of Chinese medicine dating back more than 4,000 years. It is like acupuncture—but without needles: The fingertips or thumbs apply pressure to acupoints located on the body. The system is based on the theory of qi (a form of life energy believed to flow along invisible channels, or "meridians" (see diagram, right), linking all body parts and functions so that the whole body works as an integrated unit. If the flow of qi is altered—either blocked, too weak, or too strong—it may give rise to ill health.

Applying pressure to acupoints stimulates and rebalances the flow of qi. There are over 360 different acupoints located along meridians all over the body (see right). Some of the most common points are described in this book. These points are easy to locate and safe to use. Each acupoint has a precise location and a specific therapeutic action. It may not be near the problem area.

When applying this technique, try the following:
- Before starting, find a comfortable position and ensure your hands can reach the acupoint without strain. You may find it easier to rest your arm or elbow on a table.
- Spend time finding the exact location of the acupoint, using the tip of a finger or thumb. Acupoints are often found in small depressions or hollows. You may know when you have found a point because, when pressed, there may be a slight tingling or heightened sensitivity. Usually, corresponding acupoints are located on either side of the body. Work on the appropriate points on both sides of the body.
- Apply pressure with the tips of your first or second finger or thumb. Exhale as you apply pressure, and inhale as you release pressure.
- Begin with gentle pressure and gradually increase it until you feel a slight discomfort or sensitivity. Maintain a firm pressure for 20–30 seconds on the body and 5–10 seconds on the face. Release and repeat up to 6 times, as necessary. You should start to feel the initial tenderness passing as the flow of qi is balanced. Once the feeling passes, stop applying pressure. The sensation will vary with individuals, so treatment should be adapted for your own personal needs.

Points of caution
- Never apply acupressure if under the influence of drugs or alcohol.
- If you are frail, elderly, pregnant, or have high blood pressure, use only very light pressure or avoid performing acupressure altogether.
- Do not apply acupressure directly to wounds, bruises, or veins; always work around these areas. Stop at once if you feel ill or uncomfortable.

Meridians and acupoints.

Acupressure

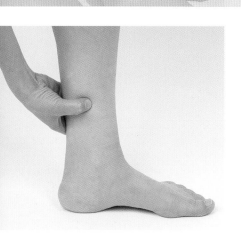

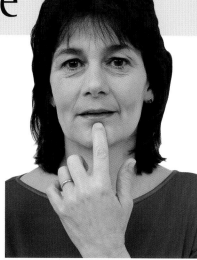

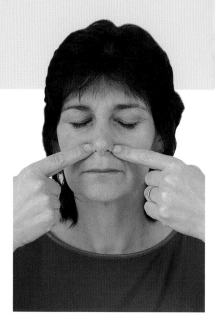

MENSTRUAL PROBLEMS

Use this acupoint to regulate menstrual problems. It is on the inside of the lower leg, 4 finger-widths above the top of the ankle bone. Apply pressure with the thumb, holding for 20–30 seconds. Repeat on other leg. Repeat daily.

TIRED FACE

This acupoint refreshes and tones facial muscles. It is located in the slight hollow in the center of the groove of the chin. Press upward slightly, using the pad of the first or second finger. Hold for 5–10 seconds. Release and repeat.

NASAL BLOCKAGE

This acupoint is located in the slight depression on the outside edges of your nostrils. Press gently with the tips of both first fingers. Hold for 5–10 seconds. Release and repeat. Use daily until the problem eases.

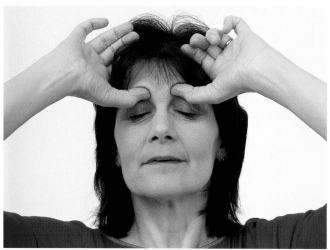

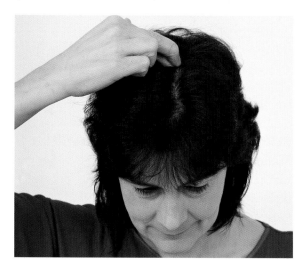

SINUSITIS AND HAY FEVER

Acupoints for alleviating the symptoms of sinusitis and hay fever are located on either side of the bridge of the nose, in the natural hollows above the inner corner of each eye, just below the inner eyebrow. Press upward with the thumbs. Hold for 5–10 seconds. Release and repeat. Use these points daily until the problem eases.

UNDERACTIVE IMMUNE SYSTEM

This acupoint boosts the immune system. It is on top of the head, at a point between the tips of the ears, in line with the nose. You will feel a slight hollow, which may be a little sensitive to touch. Apply pressure with the tip of one finger. Hold for 10–20 seconds. Release and repeat.

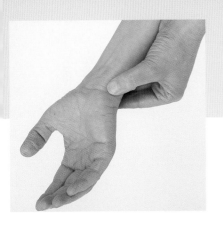
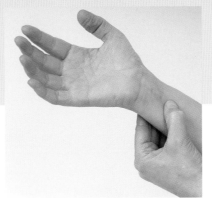
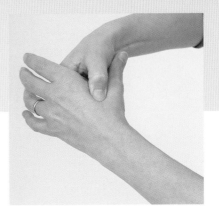

ANXIETY AND RESTLESSNESS
Use this acupoint when you need to calm your mind. It is located in a small hollow on the inner wrist, in line with the little finger. Apply pressure with the tip of a thumb pointing toward the little finger. Hold for 20–30 seconds, release, and repeat. Repeat on other wrist.

MOTION SICKNESS
This acupoint is located on the inside of the arm, 3 finger-widths below the natural crease on your wrist. Support your outer wrist with your fingers, and apply pressure with the pad of your thumb. Hold for 20–30 seconds. Release. Repeat on the other arm.

DIGESTIVE DISORDERS
This acupoint, called the Great Eliminator, lies in the fleshy area between thumb and first finger. Place the first finger of the other hand beneath it and the thumb on top. Gently squeeze and hold for 20–30 seconds. Release and repeat. Do not use in pregnancy.

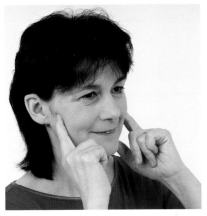
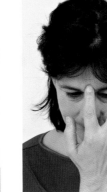
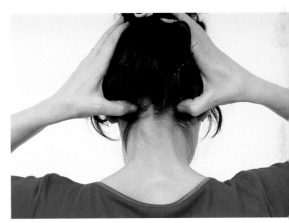

BLOCKED EARS
To find this acupoint, open your mouth a little way and feel for a slight depression in front of the ear. Close your mouth. Use your first or second finger to apply pressure toward your ear. Hold for 20–30 seconds. Release and repeat.

HEADACHE
Apply pressure, using the first or second finger, to the center of the forehead, just above the nose, and between the eyebrows. Hold for 5–10 seconds. Release. Repeat.

STIFF NECK AND TENSION HEADACHE
These acupoints lie in the slight hollows on the bony ridge at the base of the skull, on either side of the neck. Rest your thumbs on these points. Gently tilt your head back a little so the weight of your head increases pressure on your thumbs. Hold for 20–30 seconds. Release. Repeat.

EYESTRAIN
These acupoints can help relieve tired eyes and headaches and clear your vision, especially after using a computer for long periods. They are in the hollows level with the outside corners of your eyes. Apply pressure with first or second finger, angled away from the eye. Hold for 5–10 seconds. Release and repeat.

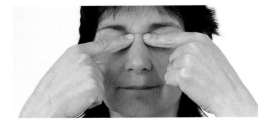

Stretching

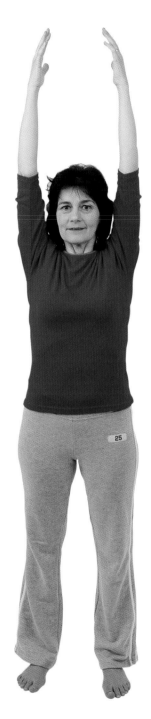

Many of the massage routines in this book include stretches. Although stretching is not a massage movement, strictly speaking, it works alongside massage and is a vital self-help technique in its own right for relieving and preventing stiffness, aches, pains, and other minor symptoms associated with our modern stressful lives.

Stretching is a natural reaction after being in one position for a long time. Think of how you desire to stretch after a long automobile journey or an afternoon spent weeding the backyard. Stretching works by taking the body in the opposite direction from the posture that you have been holding for a long time, releasing tension that has built up and keeping the body in balance.

When using this technique, try the following:
- Stretch only when your muscles are warm. An ideal time is following a warm bath or after some gentle activity.
- Keep the movement very slow and controlled. Do not force the position or bounce into a stretch.
- Stretches are held for different lengths of time. Finger stretches are usually held for around 5 seconds, while other stretches can be held for as long as 30 seconds. Stretch both sides of the body equally.
- Start very gently, and gradually build up the stretch. You should feel a slight tension that is wonderfully satisfying.
- Stretch only as far as you can without causing pain or discomfort— you will know your own limits. Overstretching, especially if you are cold, can aggravate problems. It is far more beneficial to repeat small stretches on a regular basis.
- Remember to keep breathing. Try to use breathing to help release any tension in the muscles. Exhale when you go into a stretch, and try to imagine the muscles relaxing as the air is released from your lungs. You will find this visualization really helps extend your stretch.

Raise your hands above your head for a glorious stretch that both relaxes and revives.

Try this stretch to release any tension in your upper arm and shoulder. Raise one arm and bend your elbow so that your hand reaches down your neck to your upper back. Hold your elbow with your left hand and pull gently for a count of 5. Relax and repeat on the other arm. Repeat 3 times.

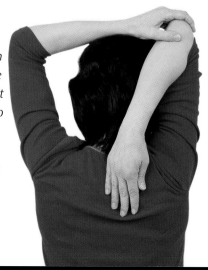

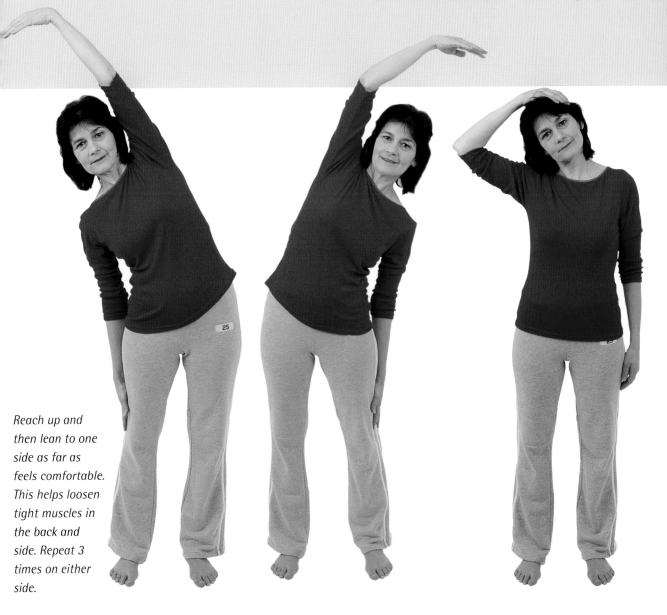

Reach up and then lean to one side as far as feels comfortable. This helps loosen tight muscles in the back and side. Repeat 3 times on either side.

Where to use

All parts of the body, from fingers to toes, can benefit from stretching. Stretching is particularly important prior to and following vigorous exercise. However, it is vital to stretch with care.

Benefits

Regular stretching will make a noticeable difference to your overall flexibility and general sense of well-being. Stretching helps maintain elasticity in the muscles that so often seem to stiffen because of poor posture or the aging process. Stretching boosts the circulation and keeps the muscles strong and supple so they function better and have more resistance to injury. Stretches also stimulate the flow of synovial fluid, which is important for lubricating the joints, thus improving and maintaining a good range of movement.

Allow your head to lean to one side to give a gentle stretch in the muscles on the other side of the neck. Stretch both sides equally to promote flexibility and balance.

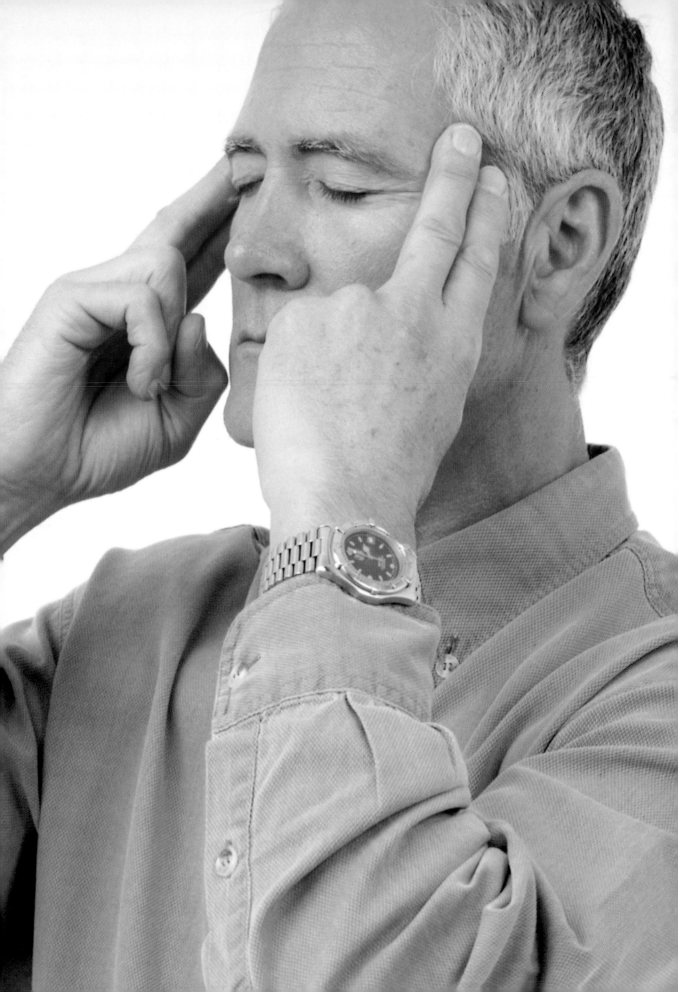

4 AT HOME

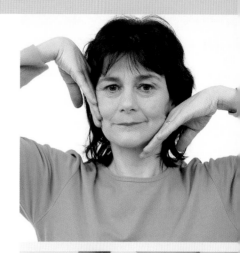

These self-massage sequences have been compiled for you to enjoy in the privacy of your own home. Try to create a restful ambience. Put on quiet music or a relaxation CD, turn down the lighting, or enjoy the gentle glow of candlelight. Wear something loose and comfortable that allows you to move easily.

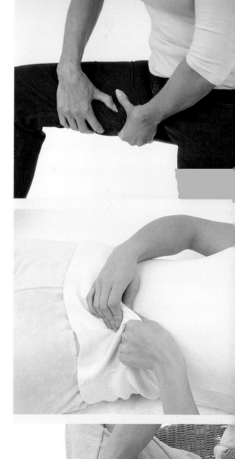

Sore feet

Try this refreshing 5–10 minute routine when your feet ache at the end of a long day. You can use a foot cream if you wish (be sure to massage over a towel), but the strokes are effective over panty hose or socks, too. You need to be able to reach your foot easily, so sit on the floor or on a chair or bed.

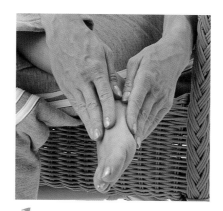

1 Start with your right foot; then work on your left. Sandwich the foot between the palms of your hands, and rub briskly so that one hand goes forward as the other goes back in short, stimulating moves. Rub for as long as feels comfortable, covering the whole foot, including the toes, heel, and ankle. Keep your hands moving so they do not stay in the same spot for too long.

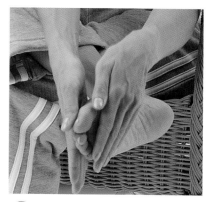

2 Sandwich your foot between the palms of your hands, and use both hands to stroke from the toes to the heel in a single continuous movement, molding your hands to the contours of your foot. Repeat as many times as you wish.

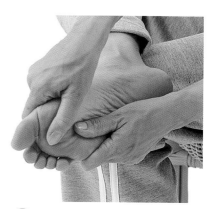

3 Now ease the tension in the sole of your foot. Support it in both hands, with your thumbs on the soles and your fingers on top. Use the pads of your thumbs to make small, firm, circular movements over the whole of your sole and around your heel. As you work, use a deep but comfortable pressure.

TOP TIPS

◆ To help relieve any aches in the arch of your foot, place a soft ball, orange, or can of soda (try it cold from the refrigerator) under the ball of your foot and roll it backward and forward for 1 minute. Repeat with the other foot.

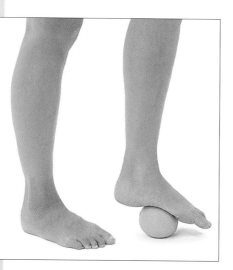

TECHNIQUE CHECKLIST

◆ Stroking ◆ Rubbing ◆ Stretching (see pages 38–55)

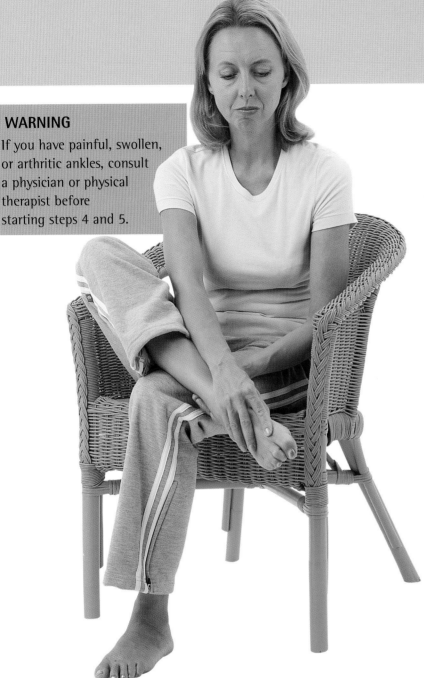

WARNING

If you have painful, swollen, or arthritic ankles, consult a physician or physical therapist before starting steps 4 and 5.

4 Rotations help ease any stiffness in the ankle. Support your leg with one hand placed just above the ankle. Clasp your foot with your other hand; then rotate your ankle in a clockwise direction. Keep the movement deliberate and controlled. Repeat 5 times in one direction and then 5 times in the other.

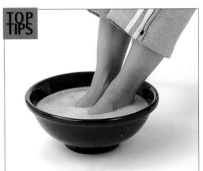

TOP TIPS

◆ For a relaxing foot soak, fill a large bowl with ankle-deep warm water. Add a few drops of mild shampoo or bath lotion. Put both feet in the foot soak and enjoy the pleasant soothing sensation for 3–5 minutes. Remove your feet from the water and dry them thoroughly.

5 Next work on your toes. Hold your foot firmly around the arch with one hand and use the other to massage each toe in turn. Rotate the toe slowly 3 times in one direction and then 3 times in the other. Finish with a gentle pull.

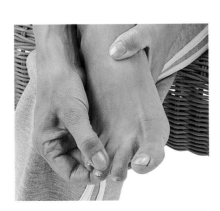

Coughs and colds

With so many germs around causing coughs and colds, you need a healthy immune system to protect you from infection. This 5-minute massage stimulates your body's defense mechanisms. The moves can be performed sitting or standing.

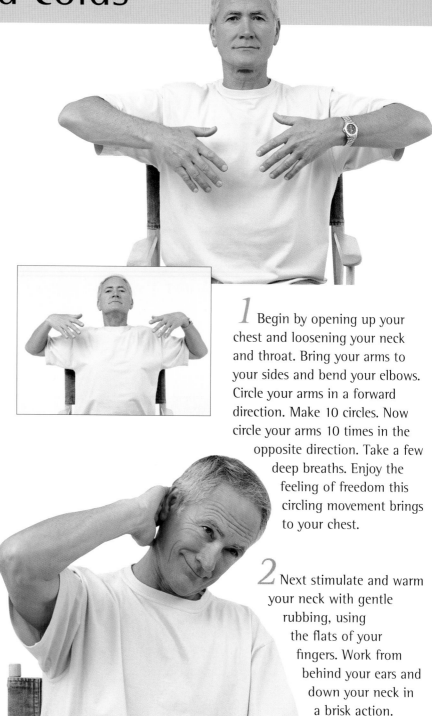

1 Begin by opening up your chest and loosening your neck and throat. Bring your arms to your sides and bend your elbows. Circle your arms in a forward direction. Make 10 circles. Now circle your arms 10 times in the opposite direction. Take a few deep breaths. Enjoy the feeling of freedom this circling movement brings to your chest.

2 Next stimulate and warm your neck with gentle rubbing, using the flats of your fingers. Work from behind your ears and down your neck in a brisk action.

TECHNIQUE CHECKLIST

◆ Stretching ◆ Rubbing ◆ Stroking ◆ Tapping ◆ Raking (see pages 38–55)

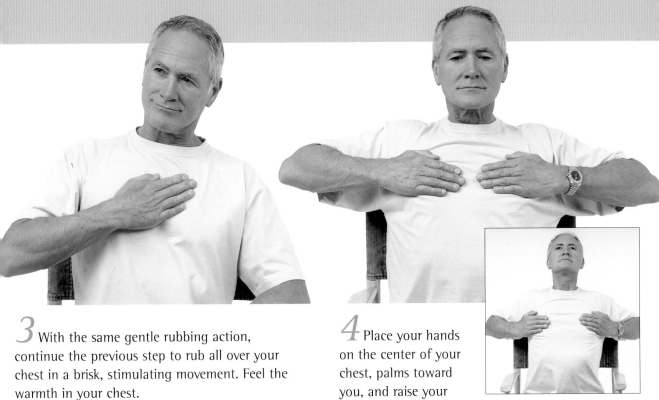

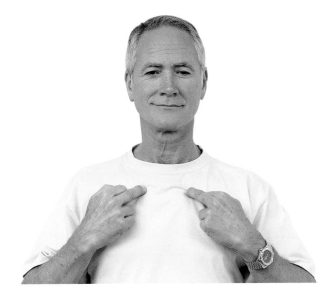

3 With the same gentle rubbing action, continue the previous step to rub all over your chest in a brisk, stimulating movement. Feel the warmth in your chest.

4 Place your hands on the center of your chest, palms toward you, and raise your elbows to your sides. Stroke from the center of your chest to your armpits. Repeat 5 times.

TOP TIPS

◆ Boost your immunity to infection by eating plenty of foods rich in vitamin C and zinc. Eat citrus fruits, strawberries, melon, kiwi fruit, green vegetables, whole grains, and seafood.

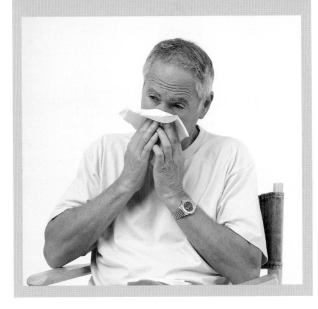

5 Now work a little deeper using the pads of one or more fingers to make fairly firm circular strokes, working from the center of your chest outward. →

Coughs and colds...continued

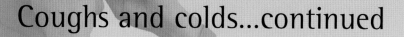

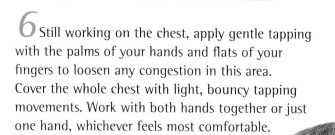

7 Soothe the area with stroking. Place the heel of your right hand on the center of your chest and sweep with a comfortable pressure toward your left armpit. Cover the whole of the left side of your chest with these strokes, gradually reducing the pressure. Change hands and repeat on the other side.

6 Still working on the chest, apply gentle tapping with the palms of your hands and flats of your fingers to loosen any congestion in this area. Cover the whole chest with light, bouncy tapping movements. Work with both hands together or just one hand, whichever feels most comfortable.

TOP TIPS

◆ During the day, drink ginger tea to soothe a sore throat and boost the body's natural defenses. (Avoid having ginger too close to bedtime, as it is very stimulating and can cause sleeping difficulties.)

8 Move your hands to your cheeks. Use the flats of your fingers to lightly but briskly rub your cheeks, jawline, and the sides of your nose. Use one or both hands, whichever feels most comfortable.

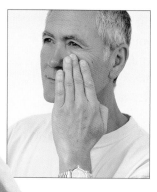

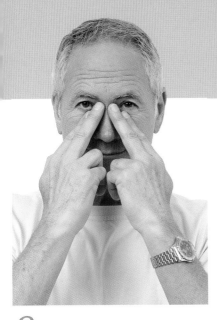

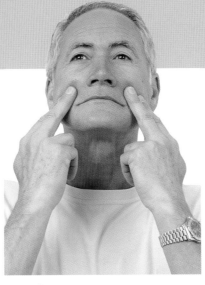

9 Place your first and second fingers on either side of the bridge of your nose and make small circular movements down each side and along your cheekbones, finishing at the sides of your ears. Repeat.

10 With hands held in the same position, stroke with a gentle pressure down your nose and along your cheekbones to your ears. Be careful not to drag the skin. Return to the starting position and repeat 5 times.

TOP TIPS

◆ Try a steam inhalation at the first hint of a cough or cold to help fight off germs. If you suffer nasal congestion, a steam inhalation helps relieve that blocked-up feeling. Add 2 drops of eucalyptus essential oil to a bowl of boiled water. Put a towel over your head, close your eyes, and inhale deeply. Stay like this for up to 10 minutes. Repeat 2–3 times a day. CAUTION: Avoid steam inhalations if you suffer from asthma.

11 Place both hands in a cupped position on your head and rake over your scalp using the pads of your fingers. With both hands working at the same time, make a long raking movement traveling over the back of your head, down your neck, and then across your chest. Repeat 5 times.

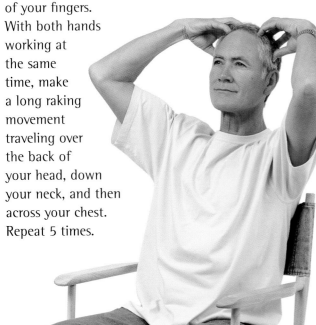

12 Finish the immune-boosting sequence with circular stroking movements over the chest, using the palms and flats of the fingers of one hand. Continue for as long as you wish.

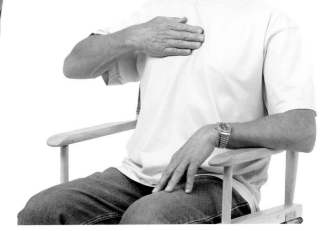

Insomnia

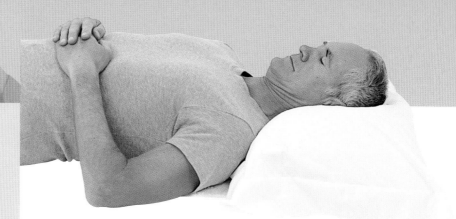

This technique, called progressive relaxation, releases tension and aids restful sleep. Before you begin, ensure that you are warm and comfortable. Lie on your back with your head supported by a small pillow, feet a little way apart, and hands by your sides. Tuck in your chin to release any tension in your neck.

The whole sequence takes around 10–15 minutes. It involves deliberately tensing and relaxing sets of muscles in sequence. Inhale as you tense the muscle and exhale as you relax.

1 Close your eyes. Be aware of the weight of your body supported by the bed. Bring your hands to rest on your abdomen. Feel their warmth radiating through your body. Now turn your attention to your breathing and try to slow down each breath. Notice how your hands rise and fall as you breathe.

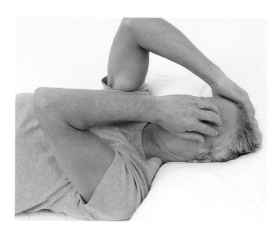

2 Take your hands to your forehead and gently stroke with a featherlike pressure over your forehead and through your hair. One hand starts the move as the other finishes in a reassuringly repetitive rhythm. Continue for as long as feels good.

3 Tense the muscles in your right foot by drawing your toes toward you. Hold for a couple of seconds and release. Repeat. Stretch your toes away from you. Hold for a couple of seconds and release. Repeat. Repeat with the left foot. Press the backs of your knees down into the bed. Hold and release. Repeat. Tense and relax buttocks, then abdomen.

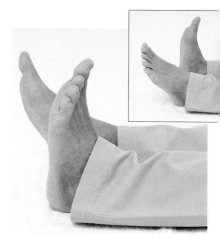

TECHNIQUE CHECKLIST

◆ Holding ◆ Stretching ◆ Feathering (see pages 38–55)

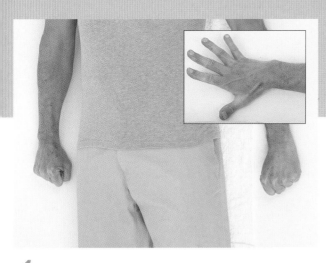

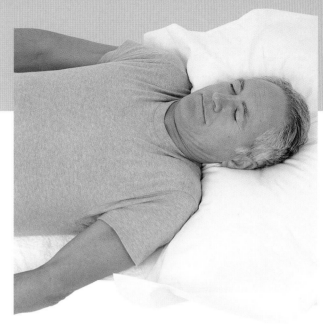

4 Make fists with both hands. Clench your fists as tightly as you can. Hold and release. Repeat. Spread your fingers apart as wide as possible. Hold this stretch for a couple of seconds and then release. Repeat.

5 Raise your shoulders. Hold for a few seconds, and then allow them to drop and relax. Repeat. Press the back of your head firmly down onto your pillow. Hold for a few seconds and release.

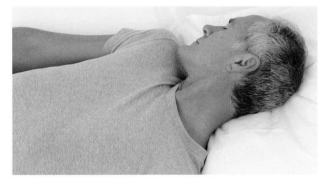

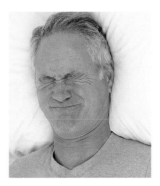

7 Tense your eyes, cheeks, and mouth muscles. Hold for a few seconds and release. Raise your eyebrows, hold for a few seconds, and release. Repeat. Enjoy the "soft" feeling in your face muscles.

6 Roll your head gently from side and side. Your neck should feel well supported by the pillow. Do not raise your head from the bed.

TOP TIPS

◆ An alternative to tensing and relaxing the muscles is to imagine the warmth and radiance of a soft light. As you focus on each set of muscles, visualize the light and feel it spreading gently through the area, relaxing and warming the muscles. Or you can just say to yourself, "Relax and let go," as you concentrate on each set of muscles.

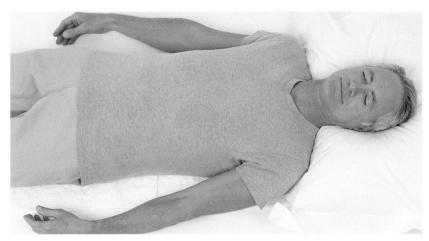

8 If you are still awake, relish the sense of relaxation and peace. Be still. Concentrate on the ebb and flow of your smooth, even breathing.

Weary legs

Self-massage is great for tired legs. Our legs support us all day long, so it's hardly surprising that they start to ache after hours of walking or standing. This 10-minute massage routine helps to relax tight muscles and boost sluggish circulation, thus reenergizing the whole body.

Use firm, upward strokes to encourage the flow of blood and lymph back to the heart. You may find this massage easier if you prop your leg on a chair or stool: Follow the massage sequence on one leg and then repeat on the other.

1 Begin by massaging your thigh. Stroke firmly from your knee to the top of your thigh with alternate hands in a rhythmic flowing motion. Use the flats of your hands and cover the front, back, and sides of the thigh.

2 Now knead the flesh of your thigh between thumbs and fingers in an alternate squeezing-and-releasing movement, one hand moving after the other. Work from your knee to the top of your thigh. Keep the pressure firm but comfortable. Work the inner and outer thigh. When your hand reaches your buttock, skim down the sides of your thigh to start again.

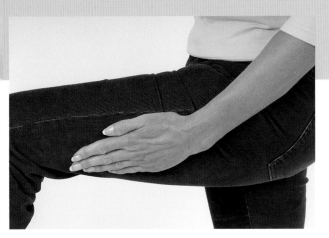

3 With the flat of one hand, rub briskly all over your thigh and buttock. Keep your hand and fingers fairly rigid to create a friction movement that encourages the healthy circulation of blood and lymph. Keep your hand moving so you do not work over the same area for too long.

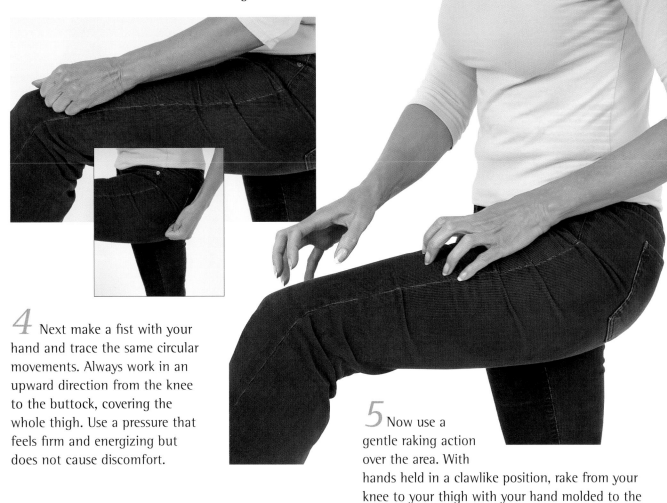

4 Next make a fist with your hand and trace the same circular movements. Always work in an upward direction from the knee to the buttock, covering the whole thigh. Use a pressure that feels firm and energizing but does not cause discomfort.

5 Now use a gentle raking action over the area. With hands held in a clawlike position, rake from your knee to your thigh with your hand molded to the contours of your leg. ➤

Weary legs...continued

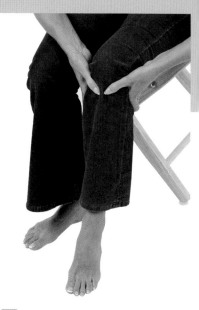

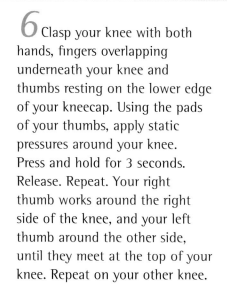

6 Clasp your knee with both hands, fingers overlapping underneath your knee and thumbs resting on the lower edge of your kneecap. Using the pads of your thumbs, apply static pressures around your knee. Press and hold for 3 seconds. Release. Repeat. Your right thumb works around the right side of the knee, and your left thumb around the other side, until they meet at the top of your knee. Repeat on your other knee.

7 With hands as before and the same pathway, massage around the sides of your knee with small circular rotations, finishing with thumbs meeting centrally above the knee. Keep your fingers at the back of the knee for support. Start with light pressure and slowly increase until firm, without causing soreness. Repeat 3 times.

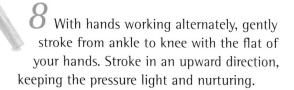

8 With hands working alternately, gently stroke from ankle to knee with the flat of your hands. Stroke in an upward direction, keeping the pressure light and nurturing.

TECHNIQUE CHECKLIST

◆ Stroking ◆ Kneading ◆ Rubbing ◆ Raking (see pages 38–55)

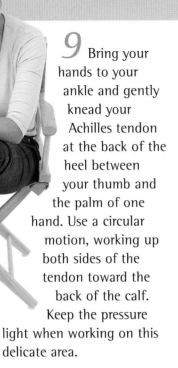

9 Bring your hands to your ankle and gently knead your Achilles tendon at the back of the heel between your thumb and the palm of one hand. Use a circular motion, working up both sides of the tendon toward the back of the calf. Keep the pressure light when working on this delicate area.

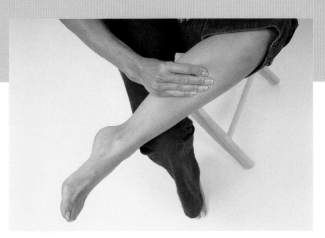

10 To loosen any tightness in your calf muscle, continue this kneading action, working in an upward direction toward your knee. When your hand reaches your knee, glide it lightly down to your ankle. Change hands and repeat over a different area of your calf muscle. Repeat 3 times.

11 Finish by stroking from your ankle up the length of your leg, moving one hand after the other or simultaneously. Start firmly, and gradually reduce the pressure until it becomes a featherlike stroke.

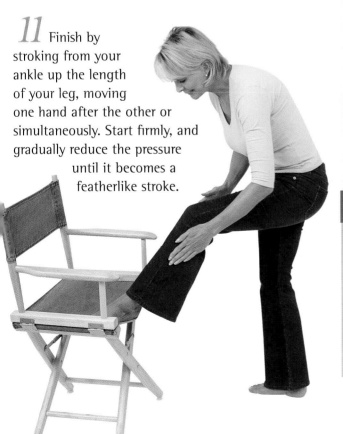

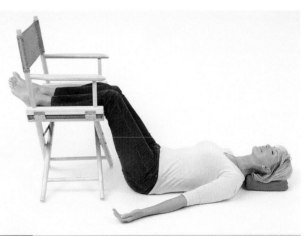

TOP TIPS

◆ If you have to stand for long periods of time, whenever you get the chance, reduce the risk of varicose veins and swelling by lying on the floor with your arms by your sides. Place your feet and lower legs on a chair so they are above your hips. Support your head and neck with a rolled towel or pillow. Rest like this for 10–20 minutes.

Hangover

A throbbing head and waves of nausea are classic symptoms of overindulgence. Of course, the best way to avoid a hangover is to moderate your alcohol intake in the first place, but if the "morning after" dawns, try this 3-minute sequence to clear your head and boost your energy levels.

This exercise is best performed sitting down but is also effective while propped up on pillows in bed.

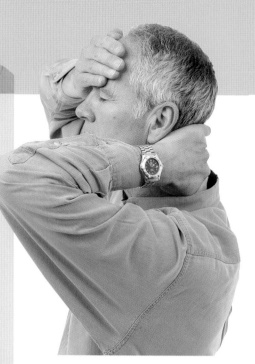

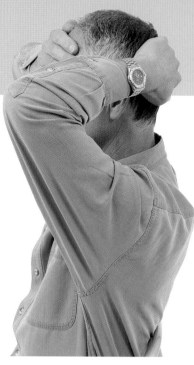

1 Place one hand on your forehead for support. Using the palm of your other hand, gently caress the back of your neck with very slow, circular, stroking movements. Continue for as long as feels good.

2 With one hand still on your forehead, bring the other one behind your head. Gently press, using as much pressure as feels comfortable. Hold for a count of 10. Release and repeat all over your head.

3 Stroke lightly through your hair with fingers relaxed and slightly splayed. At the end of each stroke, grasp some hair between your fingers and tug very gently. Release and draw your hand slowly through the tips of your hair. Repeat over front, sides, and back.

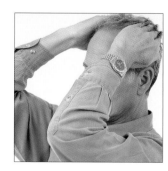

TECHNIQUE CHECKLIST

◆ Stroking ◆ Holding (see pp.38–55)

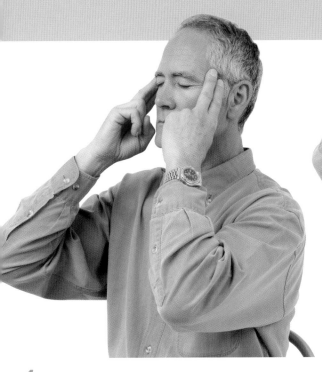

4 Now bring your hands to your temples and use the pads of 2 fingers to make light, circular pressures. Keep the movements very slow and nurturing. Continue for as long as you wish.

5 Finish with featherlike strokes, using the pads of your fingers over your forehead, working from the center to your ears. Your hands work alternately in a slow, steady rhythm.

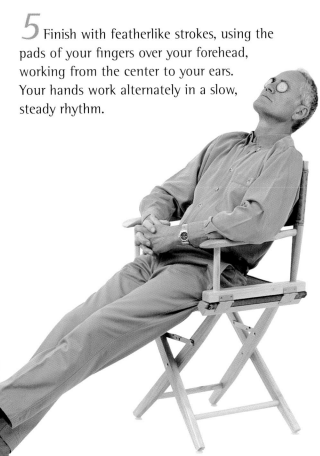

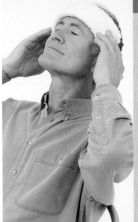

TOP TIPS

◆ A compress soothes sore heads. Add 1 drop of lavender or rosemary pure essential oil to a bowl of cold water. Soak a cloth in the water. Wring out and place on your forehead or behind your neck. Keep in place for as long as feels comfortable.

◆ Take a hot shower. Place 2 drops of rosemary pure essential oil on a facecloth or shower mitt and rub vigorously all over to revitalize mind and body.

To maximize the benefits of this sequence, soak cotton pads in cold water and place over your eyes or use slices of cool cucumber.

Constipation

Constipation is often linked to diet, stress, and tension. Eat lots of fruit and vegetables, drink plenty of fluid each day, and allow time for exercise and relaxation. If you continue to suffer occasional bouts of mild constipation, massaging your abdomen can help to stimulate the bowel and offer relief.

This sequence takes about 10 minutes and is best performed lying on your back on a comfortable surface. You can massage directly on your skin or through clothes, as you prefer. Take a few deep breaths before you begin.

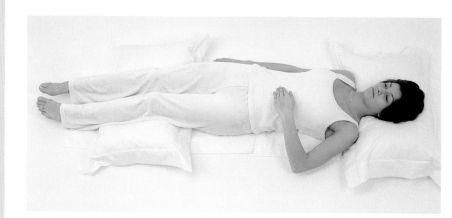

1 Place the palm of one hand (right or left) on your abdomen. Trace a small clockwise circle around your navel, using the flats of your fingers. Start with a fairly light pressure, and gradually increase the pressure so that it is firm yet comfortable. Make 4 circles.

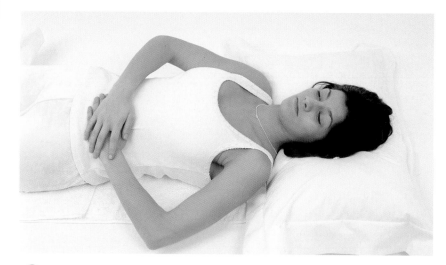

2 Now place one hand on top of the other and make larger circles using the palm of your hand, covering the whole abdominal area. Make the movement fairly firm and always in a clockwise direction to follow the path of the large intestine. Repeat 4 times.

TECHNIQUE CHECKLIST

◆ Stroking   ◆ Kneading   (see pages 38–55)

WARNING
Avoid this massage if you are pregnant or have your period unless advised otherwise by your physician.

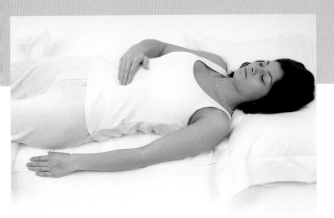

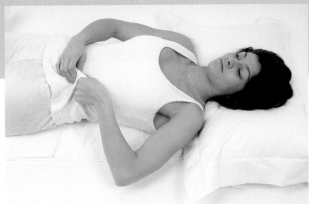

3 Use the pads of the fingers of one hand to make small rotations, following the circular path of the previous move. Make the moves slow and deliberate with a firm but comfortable pressure—you will know what feels right for you. Remember, massage should never cause pain. Trace 1 circle only.

4 Now gently knead around your abdomen and waist using your thumb and first fingers. Use alternate hands to pick up and then release the flesh. Continue until you have covered the whole of the abdominal area.

TOP TIPS

◆ A compress placed on the abdomen helps to stimulate the digestive tract. Start with a hot compress and leave in place for 3 minutes. Then use a cold compress for 1 minute. Alternate hot and cold compresses for around 10 minutes. Add 1 drop of rosemary essential oil to the water.

◆ Each morning, take time to drink a glass of fruit juice or cup of fennel or chamomile tea to encourage the natural movement of the bowel.

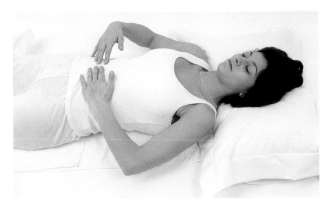

5 Calm the area with some gentle strokes working from the left side of the waist to the right side, one hand following the other in a wavelike motion. Continue for as long as you wish.

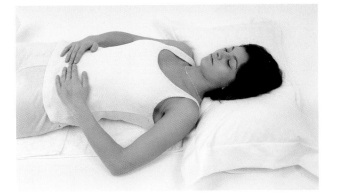

TOP TIPS

◆ Help relax your bowel by getting into the squatting position before going to the bathroom. Practice by holding on to a stable piece of furniture and lowering your hips while keeping your feet flat on the ground. This is great for toning leg muscles, too!

6 Finish the sequence by placing your palms, fingers pointing toward each other, just below your navel. Hold for a minute. Breathe slowly and deeply. Release.

Premenstrual syndrome (PMS)

Many women suffer from premenstrual syndrome (PMS) in the second half of the menstrual cycle. Symptoms vary but may include tender breasts, irritability, tearfulness, stomach cramps, puffiness, and lower–back pain.

This 10-minute sequence may not ease all of your symptoms, but it can help lift your mood and stroke away nagging aches in your back and abdomen. Keep the pressure light and gentle with plenty of repetitions.

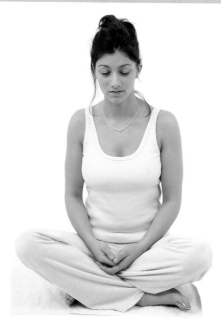

1 Begin the massage by sitting on the floor. Place your hands in your lap and breathe deeply and slowly. As you breathe in, imagine you are absorbing a deep pink light, rising up from your toes and moving through your whole body, making you feel soft and feminine. As you breathe out, try to expel any tension and negative thoughts.

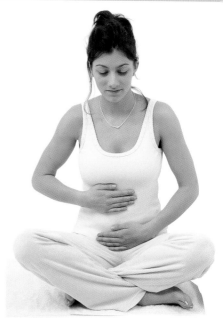

2 Place one hand on your solar plexus, in the triangle formed by the bottom ribs. Rest the flat of your other hand just below the navel. Sit quietly for 2 or 3 minutes, breathing with a normal rhythm.

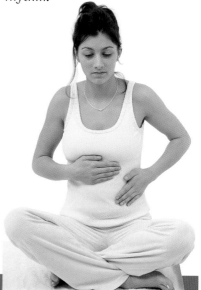

3 With your left hand still on your solar plexus, use the flat of your right hand to trace 10 gentle circles around your navel.

TECHNIQUE CHECKLIST

◆ Acupressure ◆ Holding ◆ Stroking ◆ Kneading ◆ Feathering ◆ Stretching (see pages 38–55)

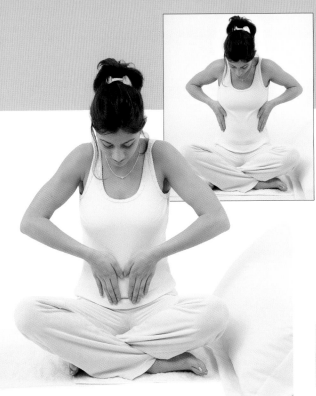

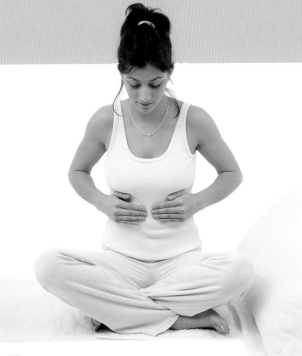

4 Place the flats of both hands on your abdomen, fingers pointing down. Bring your hands upward and then away from each other, in an outward circular movement. Your hands meet again at the bottom of the circle and continue to form 2 separate circles. Repeat as often as you wish.

5 Trace the same path with your hands as in Step 4, this time making gentle circular moves with the pads of your fingertips.

TOP TIPS

◆ To maximize the benefits of this exercise sequence massage on bare skin using 1 teaspoon (5ml) of evening primrose oil. Many women also find relief from premenstrual symptoms by supplementing their diet with evening primrose oil in capsule form, available from health food stores or your local pharmacy.

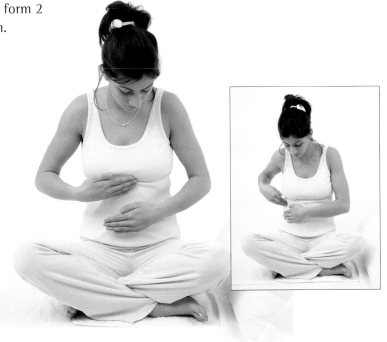

6 Stroke the whole area with a featherlike pressure. Your hands move slowly and lightly in an upward direction, working alternately or at the same time, whichever feels best for you. ➔

Premenstrual syndrome...continued

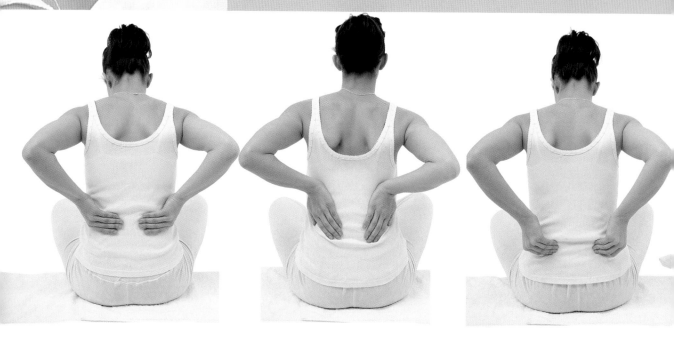

7 Bring your hands to either side of your waist with thumbs pointing toward your abdomen and fingers resting on your lower back. With the flats of your fingers, make light circular strokes all over your lower back. Continue for as long as feels good. Stretch only as far as you can comfortably reach.

8 With hands placed on either side of the spine and fingertips pointing downward, slide your hands firmly down the lower back to your buttocks. If you find it more comfortable, use the backs of your hands. Repeat 3 times.

9 Use the pads of the fingertips to work a little deeper into any areas of tension in your lower back. Find trouble spots, and ease them away with gentle kneading.

TOP TIPS

◆ Premenstrual syndrome symptoms may be exacerbated by drinking too many stimulants, such as tea, coffee, cola, and alcohol, so try limiting your intake and substituting mineral waters and herbal teas. Chamomile tea is especially calming and soothing.

10 Soothe your back with alternate hand stroking. Use the flats of your hands (or the backs of your hands if that is more comfortable) to stroke up from your buttocks to your waist, one hand moving after the other to cover the whole area.

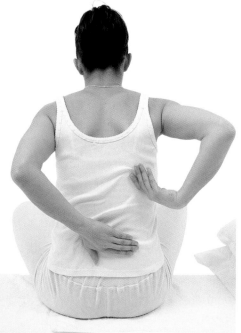

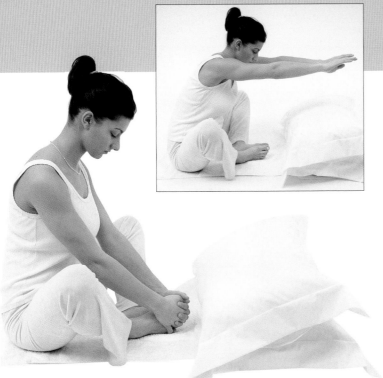

11 Bring the soles of your feet together and hold them with your hands. Take a deep breath in and then breathe out, and bend forward as far as you can comfortably reach. Hold the stretch for a count of 5, breathing normally.

12 Slowly sit up and take a few deep breaths. Cross your ankles. Raise your arms above your head and slowly circle them 3 times to ease any tension in your shoulders.

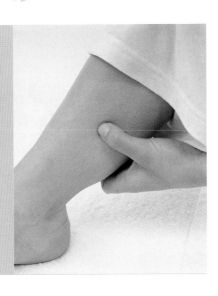

TOP TIPS

◆ An acupoint linked with alleviating PMS and period pain is located on the inside of the lower leg. Feel for the slight hollow 4 finger-widths above the top of the ankle bone. Apply pressure with your thumb. Hold for about 20–30 seconds. Release and repeat. Repeat on other leg.

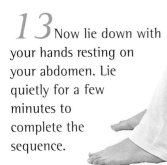

13 Now lie down with your hands resting on your abdomen. Lie quietly for a few minutes to complete the sequence.

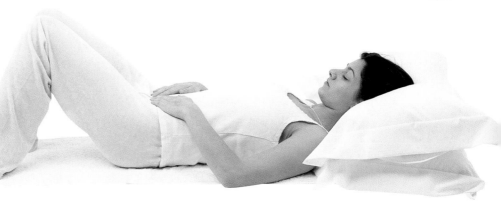

Pregnancy

During pregnancy it is especially important to look after your health to prepare for the exciting changes ahead. This routine is designed to relax the mind and strengthen both mind and body during this time. Allow 30 minutes for the routine.

Take time doing each step, and use this opportunity to focus on breathing. Use an exercise mat or folded blanket and have lots of pillows handy, as you may need them for support.
CAUTION: Always check with your doctor before doing any exercise routine.

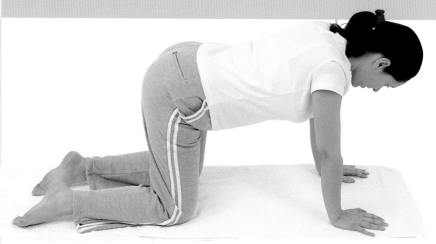

1 Begin by kneeling on the floor on your hands and knees. Place your hands shoulder width apart, arms and thighs in a vertical position. Now gently swing your hips forward and backward several times. Continue for as long as feels comfortable. You may also like to try rotating your hips or rocking them from side to side. This helps release the tension that so often builds up in the lower back during pregnancy.

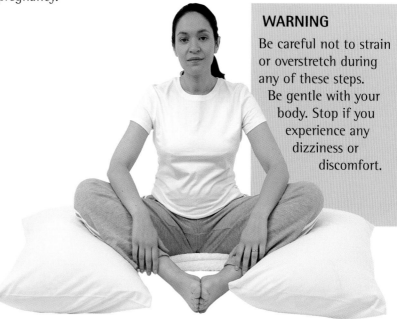

WARNING
Be careful not to strain or overstretch during any of these steps. Be gentle with your body. Stop if you experience any dizziness or discomfort.

2 Now sit on the floor with your back supported by pillows or a wall. Bend your knees and bring the soles of your feet together. Rest your knees on pillows if this feels more comfortable. Sit in this position for as long as feels comfortable. Concentrate on slowing down your breathing. Feel the release of tension in your pelvic area.

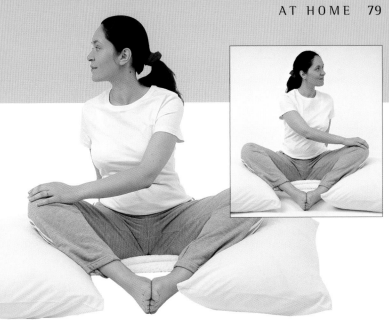

3 Now turn slowly to your right, resting your left hand on your right knee. Look over your right shoulder. Return to the center and repeat the move turning to the left. Repeat the sequence. Stop this stretch if it causes any discomfort in your lower back.

4 Place your feet on the floor with knees bent. If you are able to reach your ankles, gently massage around each ankle in turn. Use the pads of your fingers or thumbs in a gentle kneading action to help improve circulation and reduce puffiness.

TOP TIPS

◆ It may help to support your back or sides with pillows. Try different positions to find what's best for you.

◆ Gently massage your abdomen (see Step 10) using 1 teaspoon (5 ml) of mixed jojoba and sweet almond oil to moisturize your skin and enhance its elasticity.

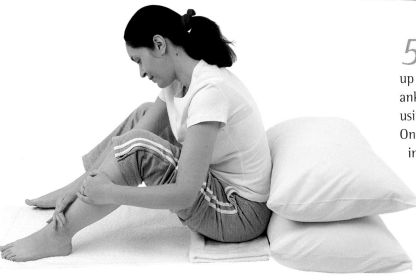

5 With knees still bent, stroke up your lower right leg from ankle to knee with long sweeps, using the palms of your hands. One hand moves after the other in a slow rhythmical action. Stroke up the front, sides, and back of your lower leg to help boost circulation and reduce the risk of varicose veins. Repeat on your left leg. →

Pregnancy...continued

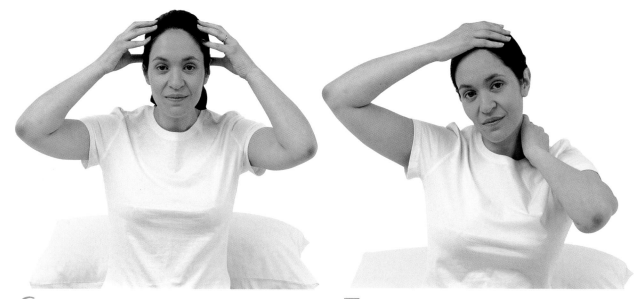

6 Bring your hands up to your head. With hands held like claws, use the pads of your fingers to make small circular pressures over your scalp. Use a gentle pressure, and keep your fingers moving continuously so that the entire scalp is covered.

7 Using alternate hands, feather-stroke from your forehead, back over your head to your neck. Keep the pressure very light, with one hand starting the movement as the other finishes. Continue for as long as feels good.

CAUTION

In late pregnancy, you may find it uncomfortable lying on your back. You can easily perform Steps 8, 9, and 10 when lying on your side.

To lie comfortably on your side, rest your head on a pillow or cushion. Bend your top knee and place a pillow or cushion between your legs to offer support.

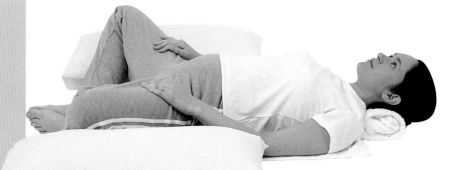

8 Now lie on your back with your head supported. Tuck your chin in to help lengthen and relax your neck. Bend your knees, bring the soles of your feet together, and allow your knees to fall gently apart. Rest for several minutes, enjoying the gentle stretch in your thighs.

TECHNIQUE CHECKLIST

◆ Stretching ◆ Kneading ◆ Stroking (see pages 38–55)

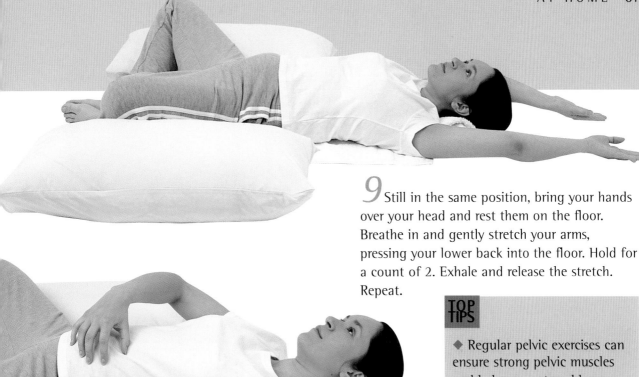

9 Still in the same position, bring your hands over your head and rest them on the floor. Breathe in and gently stretch your arms, pressing your lower back into the floor. Hold for a count of 2. Exhale and release the stretch. Repeat.

TOP TIPS

◆ Regular pelvic exercises can ensure strong pelvic muscles and help prevent problems, such as stress incontinence. An easy way is to lie on the floor with your head well supported. Bend your knees and place your feet flat on the floor. To locate your pelvic muscles, pretend you need to stop the flow of urine. Tighten these muscles and imagine you are lifting them inside you, like an elevator, stopping at different floors. Hold the squeeze for a count of 4, lift them a little farther in, hold for a count of 4. Now let the elevator go down, stopping at as many floors as you can manage.

10 Bring your hands to your abdomen and gently rake from one side to the other, one hand moving after the other in opposite directions. Keep the pressure very light and nurturing as you caress your unborn baby.

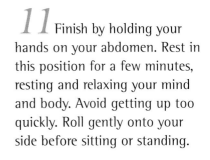

11 Finish by holding your hands on your abdomen. Rest in this position for a few minutes, resting and relaxing your mind and body. Avoid getting up too quickly. Roll gently onto your side before sitting or standing.

Menopausal mood swings

A balance of regular exercise and daily relaxation helps promote health and vitality throughout menopause and can alleviate mood swings and other symptoms. These 12 simple steps encourage you to move your body and relax your mind and can boost positive well–being.

The sequence takes 10–15 minutes, so set aside time for yourself. Dim the lights, play gentle music, and hang a DO NOT DISTURB sign on the door. This is your time. You deserve it.

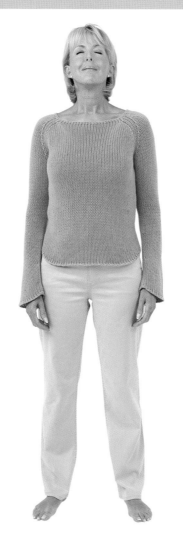

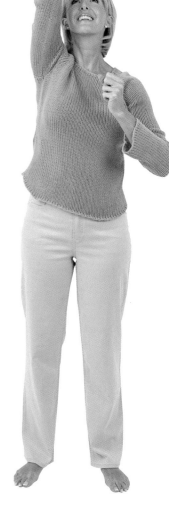

1 Stand with your hands held loosely by your sides. Then just relax. Let go of all the demands and pressures and become as floppy as a rag doll. Now shake out any tension—quite literally. Shake your head, shake your hands, shake your shoulders, shake your legs, and your whole body.

2 Lift your arms above your head and stretch up as far as you can reach in comfort. Make loose fists with your hands and punch upward, one after the other.

TOP TIPS

◆ If you find it hard to sleep at night, place 2 drops (no more) of lavender essential oil on your pillow or on a tissue tucked under your pillow.

TECHNIQUE CHECKLIST

◆ Stretching ◆ Kneading ◆ Pressures (see pages 38–55)

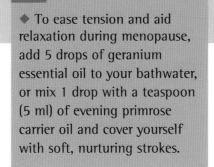

TOP TIPS

◆ To ease tension and aid relaxation during menopause, add 5 drops of geranium essential oil to your bathwater, or mix 1 drop with a teaspoon (5 ml) of evening primrose carrier oil and cover yourself with soft, nurturing strokes.

3 Place your arms in front of you. Now swing them from one side to the other, letting them move in a gentle, relaxed manner. Continue this rhythmic swaying action, gradually allowing your upper body to gently twist at the same time as your arms. Keep your head in line with your arms.

4 With your feet shoulder-width apart, bend down and cup your knees with your hands. Keep your feet on the floor and hands on your knees as you circle them 6 times in one direction and 6 times in the other.

5 Now release some of those "feel good" hormones associated with regular exercise. Begin by walking on the spot. Keep one foot in contact with the floor at all times, raising and lowering your heels in turn. Make the movement slow and deliberate. When you feel ready, begin lifting your knees to march on the spot. Increase the speed. Bring your arms into the movement too. Continue for at least 10 alternate knee lifts. →

Menopausal mood swings...continued

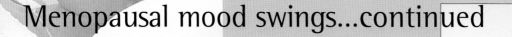

7 With your hands still held in the same position, gently knead your lower back with your fingers. Feel for any areas of tension and pay special attention to these. Continue for as long as feels good.

8 Now gently soothe away any tension in your neck. Support your forehead with one hand and bring the other hand to your neck. Use the flats of your fingers to make large, comforting circular movements over your neck and the back of your head. Complete about 6 circles.

6 Place your hands on your lower back, fingers pointing toward one another. Keep your head and shoulders still while you rotate your hips in a clockwise direction. Trace 6 circles with your hips. Enjoy the sense of freedom this flowing movement brings to the whole hip area. Repeat in the other direction.

9 Now bring both hands to your head to gently knead your scalp. In a clawlike position, make circular rotations with your fingertips all over your scalp. Feel your scalp move beneath your fingers as it starts to relax and loosen. Enjoy!

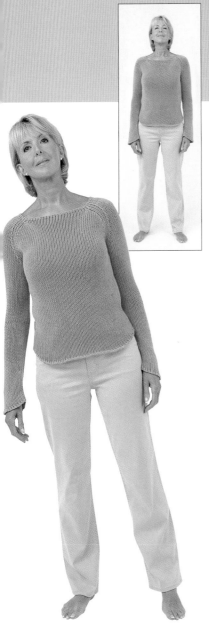

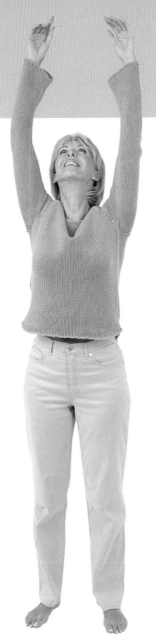

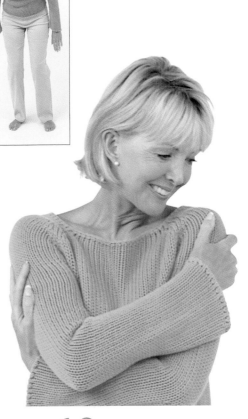

12 Finish by crossing your arms over your chest and giving yourself a big hug.

10 Bring your hands down and allow them to hang loosely by your sides. Stand tall, with back straight, shoulders relaxed, and tummy tucked in. Sway gently from one foot to the other and then stand still. Spread your toes out so you are standing on a firm base. Take a few deep breaths, in and out. Imagine the breath circulating around your whole body, filling you with a sense of lightness and peace. Stay in this quiet pose for a few minutes.

11 Take a deep breath in and then exhale as you swing your arms up and over your head. Keep your knees loose and flexible to allow freedom of movement. Stretch out your arms. Repeat 3 times.

TOP TIPS

◆ Peppermint has useful cooling properties. So if you are troubled by hot flashes, try a cup of peppermint tea. You may also find it helpful to reduce your intake of hot drinks and spicy foods. Be sure, too, to wear several layers of thin clothing so you can easily adapt to changes in temperature during the day by adding or removing items.

Puffy ankles

If your ankles often swell, try this 5-minute self-massage sequence, followed by a 20-minute rest with legs raised. This exercise is performed while sitting on a comfortable surface, such as a towel or blanket on the floor.

Do Steps 1–4 on your right leg and then repeat on your left leg. To enhance its beneficial effect and help reduce fluid retention, try the massage using 1 teaspoon (5 ml) of evening primrose oil mixed with 1 drop of geranium pure essential oil.

1 Bend your knee so that you can reach your ankle comfortably. Keep your foot flat on the floor, if possible. Stroke from your foot to your knee, using the flats of your hands. Keep the movement slow and gentle.

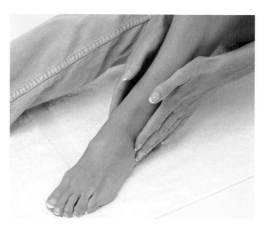

2 Now stroke around your anklebone with the pads of 2 fingers. Circle the ankle with one flowing movement, working in a clockwise direction. Make at least 6 circles. Repeat in the opposite direction. Continue for as long as feels good.

3 Next use the fleshy pads of 2 or more fingers to make small kneading rotations around your anklebone. Massage both sides of the ankle simultaneously, working in a clockwise direction. Repeat 3 times.

TECHNIQUE CHECKLIST

◆ Stroking ◆ Holding ◆ Stretching (see pages 38–55)

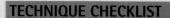

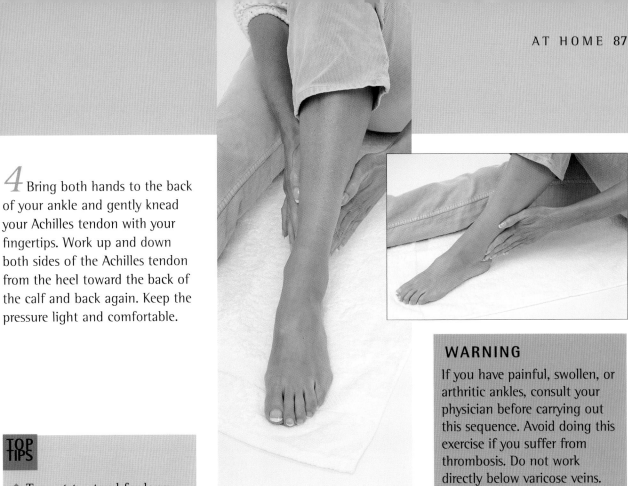

4 Bring both hands to the back of your ankle and gently knead your Achilles tendon with your fingertips. Work up and down both sides of the Achilles tendon from the heel toward the back of the calf and back again. Keep the pressure light and comfortable.

TOP TIPS

◆ Try not to stand for long periods of time. If there is no option, then contract and release your calf muscles at intervals during the day.

◆ The following foods are mild diuretics, so try including them in your diet: carrots, leeks, cucumber, watermelon. Drink lots of fluids, including lemon juice and dandelion tea.

◆ Rest your legs on pillows at the bottom of your bed while you sleep.

WARNING

If you have painful, swollen, or arthritic ankles, consult your physician before carrying out this sequence. Avoid doing this exercise if you suffer from thrombosis. Do not work directly below varicose veins.

5 Clasp your knees to your chest. With arms held under your knees to offer support, gently rotate one ankle in a clockwise direction. Keep the action definite and controlled, aiming to achieve a full range of movement without forcing the action. Repeat in both directions 5 times. Repeat with the other ankle.

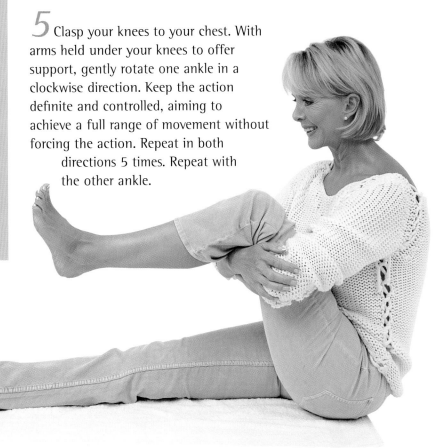

Facial lines and wrinkles

As skin ages, it starts to lose its elasticity and firmness. Massage will not reverse the aging process, but it can boost the flow of blood and lymph, adding a healthy glow and nourishing the skin and facial muscles.

Massage can also help speed the removal of toxins and waste products—which play havoc with skin texture—and tones and lifts facial muscles to give a youthful look. Try this 5-minute facelift while applying your daily moisturizer.

1 Close your eyes. Place the pads of your third fingers on the inner edge of the eyebrows. Make very small and gentle circular stroking movements, working all the way around your eyes. Glide lightly over the surface of the skin.

2 Continue these circular strokes all over your face and under your chin.

TOP TIPS

◆ Dry-brushing your facial skin helps slough off dead, dry cells and encourages a healthy, glowing appearance. However, it is important to be gentle, because the skin on your face is delicate. Use a soft, dry washcloth or a facial brush.

3 Bring your first or second fingers to your cheekbones. Gently press and then rotate the pads of your fingers so the skin moves against the bone. Be careful not to drag your skin. Lift your fingers, move to the next spot, and repeat, working along your cheekbones toward your ears. Repeat these stationary circles all over your cheeks, maintaining a very gentle pressure.

TECHNIQUE CHECKLIST

◆ Stroking ◆ Pressures ◆ Kneading ◆ Tapping (see pages 38–55)

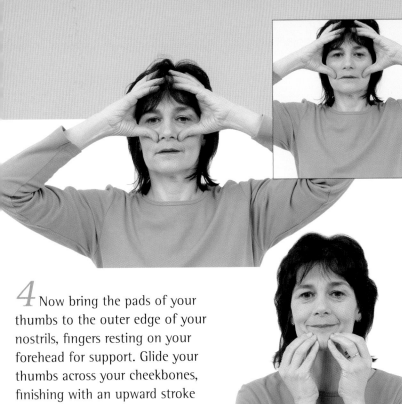

◆ A helpful acupoint for toning facial muscles and improving your complexion lies in a slight hollow in the center of the groove of your chin. Use the pad of your first or second finger to press in a slightly upward direction. Hold for 5–10 seconds. Release and repeat.

4 Now bring the pads of your thumbs to the outer edge of your nostrils, fingers resting on your forehead for support. Glide your thumbs across your cheekbones, finishing with an upward stroke to your ears. Repeat the stroking movement 3 times with your thumbs starting a little farther up your nose each time. Avoid the delicate skin under the eyes. Repeat the whole sequence.

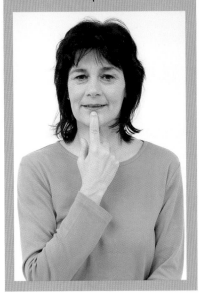

5 Place fingers above chin with thumbs underneath. Gently squeeze and rotate your fingers without moving the thumbs. Continue along your jawbone to your ears.

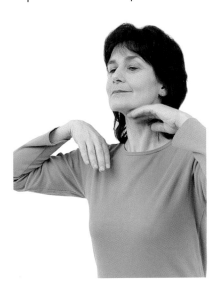

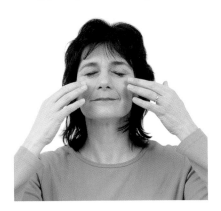

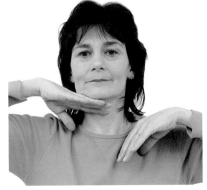

6 With palms facing downward, gently pat under your chin and around your jawline. Use alternate hands to tap in an upward, flicking action, covering the whole area.

7 Cover your face with gentle fingertip tapping to give the skin a glow. Keep the movement light and bouncy, moving rapidly over your cheeks, nose, and forehead. Include your ears if you wish.

8 Finish by stroking up from your chest to your chin with the backs of your fingertips, working in long, flowing sweeps. One hand moves after the other in a rhythmic action.

Tired face

Your face muscles are always working. And like all busy muscles, they get tense and taut. This can lead to eyestrain, and headaches, and can add years to your age.

This 5-minute massage sequence helps relax tense muscles, making your face look softer, younger, and more refreshed. Mind and body will feel more relaxed, too. An ideal time is before bed, but try it whenever you feel the cares of the world starting to show on your face.

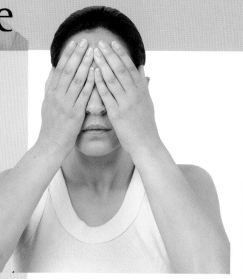

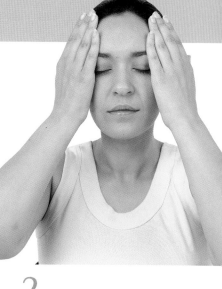

1 Cover your face with the palms of your hands, keeping fingers close together. Now gently press on your face with your hands, hold for a count of 3, and release. Repeat 3 times.

2 Move your hands up a little. Using the flats of your fingers, stroke across your forehead from the center to the sides.

3 Place your hands on your cheeks with the palms against your skin and fingers pointing upward. Keeping your hands soft and relaxed, lightly rub up and down, covering the whole of the cheek area. Your hands move over the surface of your skin without dragging it. Feel the warmth as the gentle rubbing action boosts blood circulation to your face.

TOP TIPS

◆ If your eyes are sunken or you have dark circles, it is likely that you are dehydrated. Make an effort to drink more water, herbal teas, or fresh fruit juice to restore hydration levels. Keep a bottle of water by your bed at night and drink a large glass on waking to replace fluid lost during the night.

TECHNIQUE CHECKLIST

◆ Stroking   ◆ Rubbing   ◆ Stretching   ◆ Feathering   (see pages 38–55)

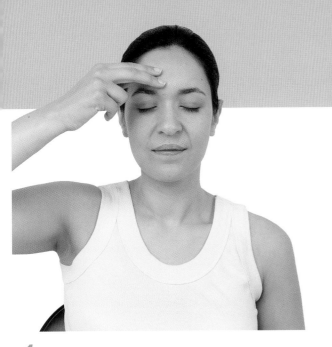

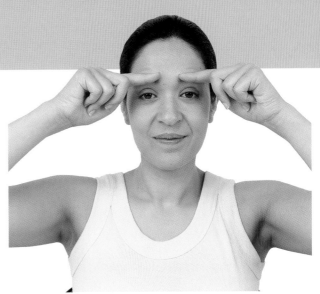

4 Place the pads of 2 or 3 fingers on the center of your forehead. This location is known as the "third eye" and is regarded as a spiritual center. With a gentle stroking movement, use your fingers to trace a circle starting at the hairline and working down to the eyebrows and back again. Repeat 3 times.

5 Place both first fingers along the length of your eyebrows, fingers pointing toward each other. Keep your eyes open and look ahead. Push your eyebrows slightly upward against the bone. Hold. Now close your eyes very slowly. Still pushing and holding, shut your eyes as tight as you can. Hold for a count of 3 and slowly release. Open your eyes and look ahead.

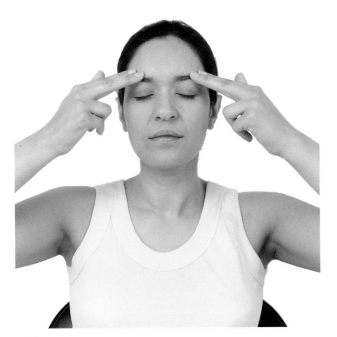

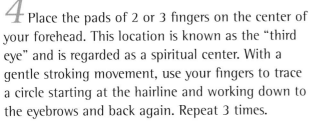

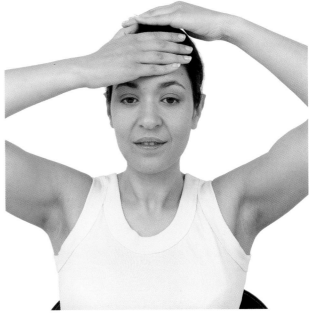

6 Make soothing circles around your eyes. Use the pads of 1 or 2 fingers to stroke along the eyebrows, starting from the center and working outward, then over the top of the cheeks and up the bridge of the nose to complete the circle. Repeat 3 times.

7 Finish by feather-stroking your forehead with the palms of your hands. Start at your eyebrows and stroke upward to the hairline. Use both hands alternately so that one stroke flows smoothly into the next. Continue for as long as you wish.

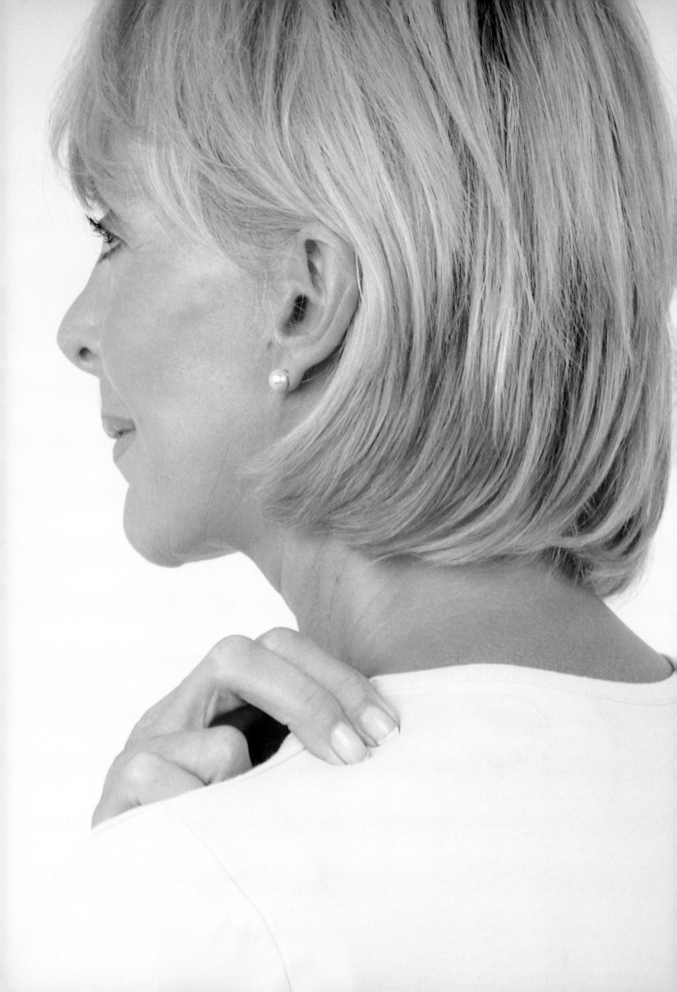

5 ON THE MOVE

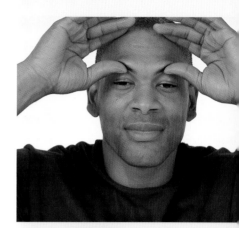

Traffic jams, crowded stations, and heavy luggage can make traveling a misery. Whether you're embarking on a long journey or simply taking a trip to the store, the following self-massage routines can take the aches and pains out of being on the move. Indeed, you may even decide to take the opportunity to relax and recharge yourself with some discreet self-massage techniques that can be done anywhere at any time. As these routines illustrate, when you are out and about, even simple movements can make all the difference, not only to your comfort but also your general health.

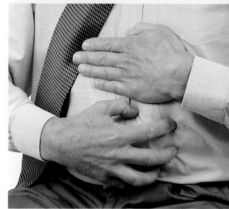

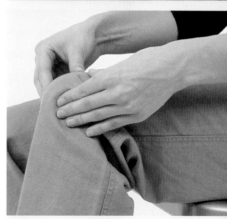

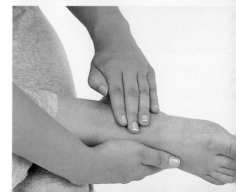

Anxiety

Breath control is an effective way of keeping your cool in times of stress. Use this 5-minute routine for relief from anxiety. The routine encourages slow, steady breathing to help you regain control of mind and body and helps bring a sense of inner peace.

Repeat the routine during quiet times to recall the sense of calm it brings when you next feel your anxiety levels rising. Depending on the circumstances, the routine can be performed wherever you are—whether sitting, standing, or lying down.

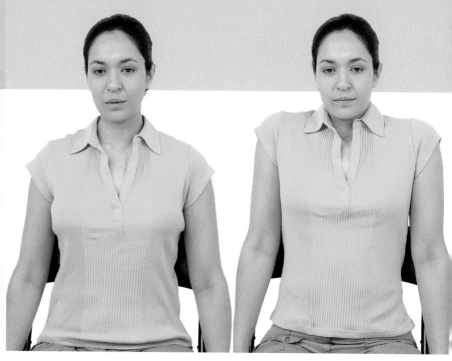

1 First concentrate on your breathing. Take in as much air as you comfortably can, either through your nose or your mouth. Then breathe out, aiming to expel all the air from your lungs. Imagine you are releasing your fears and worries.

2 On your next breath, turn your attention to your shoulders, which often become tense and tight when we feel anxious. As you breathe in, raise your shoulders. As you breathe out, release your shoulders. Feel the tension slowly dissipating.

TOP TIPS

◆ A useful acupoint for calming fear, agitation, and restlessness is located on the inside of the wrist in a small hollow in line with your little finger. Apply a firm pressure with the tip of your thumb facing toward your little finger. Hold for 20–30 seconds, release, and repeat. Repeat on the other wrist.

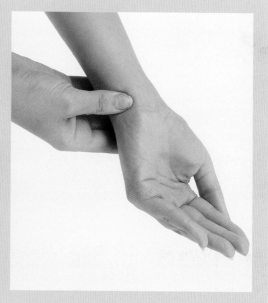

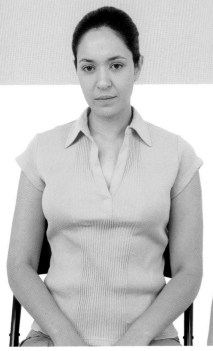

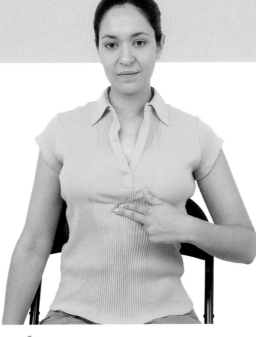

3 Concentrate on breathing out and let your shoulder muscles relax and let go of tension. It may help to say a single word as you exhale, such as "calm" or "peace." Repeat this cycle of deep breathing 3 times. Return to your normal rhythm of breathing, with shoulders remaining still as you breathe in and out.

4 Now place the fingertips of your left hand just below your breastbone. This is the solar plexus, a meeting point for a network of nerves. Holding your solar plexus helps calm and relax the whole nervous system. Hold for 2 or 3 breaths. Release and repeat. Keep your breathing slow and controlled.

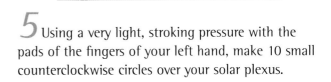

TECHNIQUE CHECKLIST

◆ Stretching   ◆ Kneading (see pages 38–55)

5 Using a very light, stroking pressure with the pads of the fingers of your left hand, make 10 small counterclockwise circles over your solar plexus.

Sinus congestion

Acute attacks of sinusitis can be very painful and need prompt medical attention. But ongoing sinus problems, such as blocked nasal passages and a dull, throbbing head, respond well to this 10-minute sequence.

The exercise combines massage with acupressure to relieve pain, ease congestion, and help prevent infection. It is also beneficial for hay fever symptoms. Do this exercise 2 or 3 times daily until the congestion and pain ease. Do not be alarmed if you notice a "popping" sensation in your head—this shows the excess mucus is starting to clear.

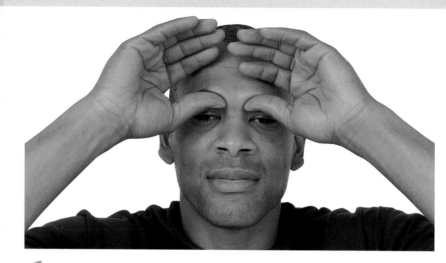

1 Press the tips of your thumbs into the acupoints (see pages 51–53) located in the small hollows on the inner edge of each eyebrow. Press upward. Hold for a count of 5 and release. Repeat. Rest your fingers on your forehead for support.

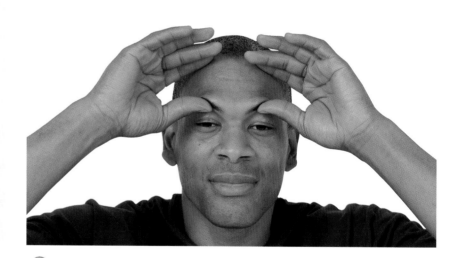

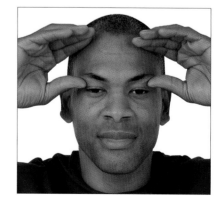

2 With your hands held in the same position, make static pressures along the ridge of each eyebrow, pushing upward against the bone. Press, hold for a count of 3, and then release. When you reach the outer edge, return to the starting position. Repeat 3 times.

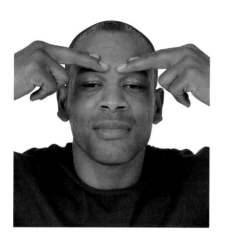

3 Smooth over your eyebrows with the pads of 2 fingers, working from the inner to the outer corners. Continue the stroking movement over your temples toward your ears. Repeat 3 times.

TOP TIPS

◆ If you are prone to sinus problems, consider reducing your intake of dairy products and foods containing wheat, since they tend to encourage the production of mucus.

4 Place both first fingers on either side of the bridge of your nose. Now make gentle circular pressures with the pads of your fingers. Release, and move to a spot a little farther down your nose. Continue these pressures down the sides of your nose toward the nostrils. Repeat 3 times.

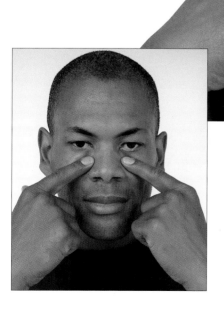

5 Using the pads of both first fingers, stroke down the sides of your nose with a firm but comfortable pressure. Repeat 3 times. →

TECHNIQUE CHECKLIST

◆ Acupressure ◆ Pressures ◆ Stroking (see pages 38–55)

Sinus congestion...continued

◆ Place 1 drop each of eucalyptus and lavender essential oils on a paper tissue and inhale deeply 2 or 3 times. Repeat 3 or 4 times during the day.

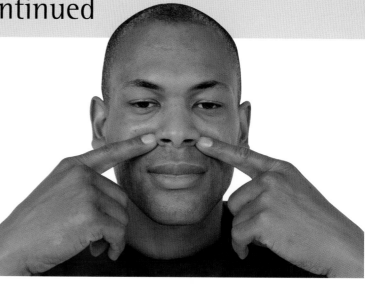

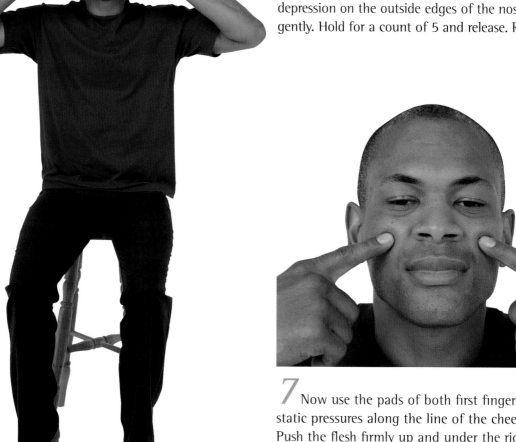

6 Place the tips of your first fingers on the acupoints (see pages 51-53) located in the slight depression on the outside edges of the nostrils. Press gently. Hold for a count of 5 and release. Repeat.

7 Now use the pads of both first fingers to apply static pressures along the line of the cheekbones. Push the flesh firmly up and under the ridge of the bones. Press, hold for a count of 3, release, and move to the next spot. Return to the starting position and repeat 3 times.

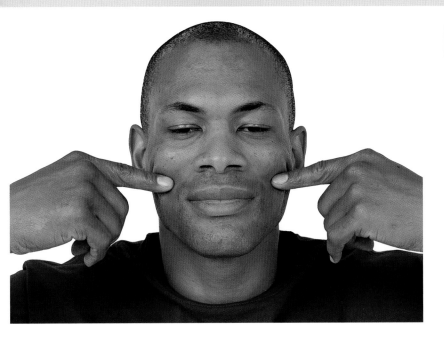

◆ Add garlic to your diet to help fight infection. Combining parsley with garlic helps reduce the odor.

◆ Use comfortably hot and cold compresses alternately on the sinus area to reduce pain. Add 1 drop of lavender pure essential oil to the water to enhance the benefits. Start with a hot compress and leave in place for 2 minutes; then use a cold compress for 1 minute. Repeat 2 or 3 times.

◆ Simply splash your face and sinuses with comfortably hot and cold water. Splash with hot water for 2 minutes, then with cold water for 1 minute. Repeat 2 or 3 times.

8 Make sweeping movements with the pads of both first fingers, following the same pathway. Release when you reach your ears. Repeat 3 times. Complete the sequence with gentle fingertip tapping all over your face and head (see page 50), especially around your sinus areas.

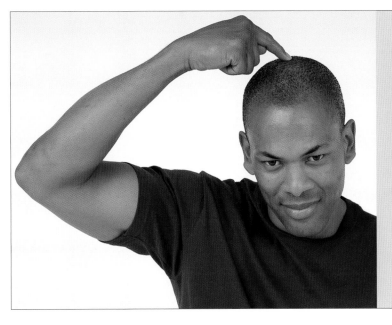

A useful acupoint for clearing your head is located on the top of your head, directly above the tips of your ears and in line with your nose. This point also helps boost the immune system (see page 52). You will feel a small hollow, which may be slightly sensitive to the touch. Apply pressure with the tip of a finger or with a fingertip placed on top of the other. Hold for a count of 10–20. Release and repeat.
CAUTION: Avoid if you have high blood pressure.

Cold hands

Cold weather often restricts blood circulation to the extremities. So if you suffer from ice-cold fingers, try this 5-minute warming sequence to bring some warmth back into your hands.

The movements are discreet, so you can try a few while sitting on the bus or standing in a line. You don't even need to take off your gloves if you don't want to.

Always wear several layers of loose, thin clothing to trap body heat, and choose mittens rather than gloves because fingers stay warmer when they're not separated.

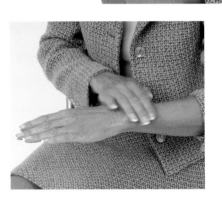

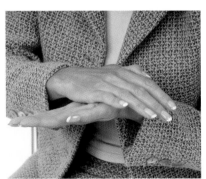

1 Begin by rubbing the back of one hand with the flat of your other hand. Rub the wrist, too. This feels wonderfully warming. Continue for as long as feels good. Switch hands and repeat.

2 Place palms together. Keep your lower hand still, and rub the palm with the heel of the other hand. Rub up and down, then in a brisk circular movement. Repeat with the other hand.

TECHNIQUE CHECKLIST

◆ Rubbing   ◆ Tapping   ◆ Stretching   ◆ Stroking   (see pages 38–55)

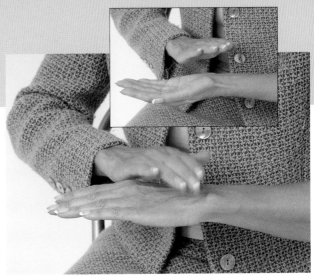

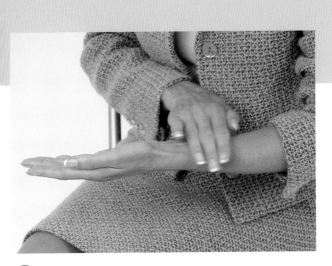

3 Again using the flat of your hand, make brisk back-and-forward rubbing movements up your inner arm from your wrist to your elbow. Turn your arm over and repeat the rubbing action, working from your fingers to your elbow.

4 Gently tap the back of your hand with the flat of your other hand. Keep your wrists flexible and allow your hand to bounce back as soon as it lands. Cover the whole hand, including the fingers and wrist. Turn your hand over and continue the springy movement across your palm, fingers, and inner wrist. Finish with some gentle stroking to soothe the area.

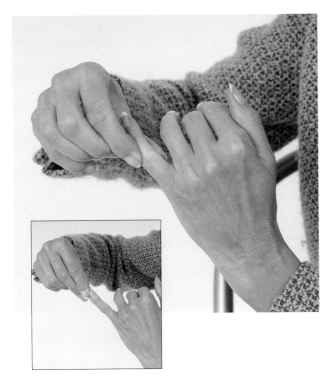

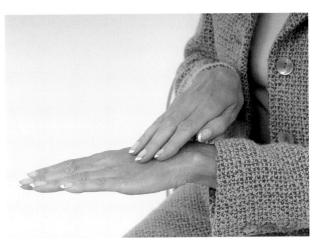

5 Grasp the little finger of one hand between the thumb and fingers of your other hand. Hold, and gently squeeze for a count of 5. Now release the pressure slightly and draw your hand along the finger, allowing it to slide off the tip in a gentle, pulling, stretching movement. Repeat. Repeat on each finger in turn, finishing with the thumb.

6 Complete the sequence by using the palm of one hand to make comfortably firm strokes along the back of your other hand. Work from your fingers to your wrist. Repeat on the other hand.

Indigestion

Rushing meals and eating on the move can cause excess gastric acid, which irritates the stomach lining, leading to heartburn and indigestion. Stress and emotional upsets can make the problem even worse.

This simple massage sequence is useful in calming the stomach and encouraging healthy digestion. You can massage through your clothes or, to enhance the benefits, remove your top and massage using 1 teaspoon (5 ml) of sunflower oil with 1 drop of lavender essential oil.

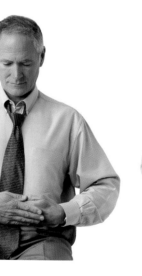

TOP TIPS

◆ To relieve indigestion, use the acupoint located in the fleshy area between thumb and forefinger called the Great Eliminator (see page 53). Place the first finger of the other hand beneath and the thumb on top. Gently squeeze and hold for 20–30 seconds. Release and repeat. CAUTION: *Do not use this acupoint in pregnancy.*

1 Sit upright in a chair. Place your hands, one on the other, on the lower abdomen, just below your navel. Hold for 1 minute.

2 Bring your hands to your navel. Make 10 small, slow, clockwise circles around your navel. Keep the pressure very gentle. Gradually increase the size and depth of the circles without interrupting the repetitive rhythm of the circular stroking. Complete about 30 circles.

TECHNIQUE CHECKLIST

◆ Stroking   ◆ Holding   ◆ Raking   (see pages 38–55)

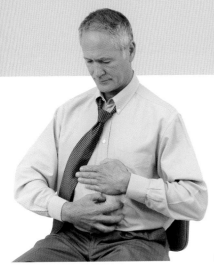

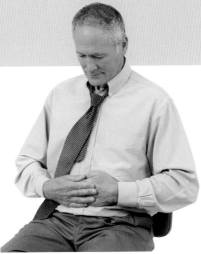

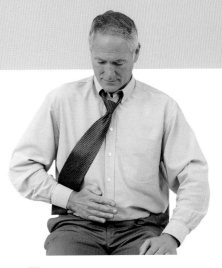

3 Hold your right hand in a wide clawlike position and trace 10 circles around your abdomen using a raking action. Always work in a clockwise direction, following the path of food as it travels along your digestive tract.

4 Now place your hands, one on top of the other, in a central position just below your rib cage. Breathe in. As you breathe out, gently vibrate your hands up and down on the same spot. Move your hands a little farther down and repeat. Make about 10 of these vibrating moves, working down to just below your navel.

5 Rest the palm of your right hand just below your rib cage on the right side of your body. Press down with the heel of your hand and stroke all the way across your abdomen to the left side. Repeat. Move your hand a little way down and repeat the sliding movement. Repeat.

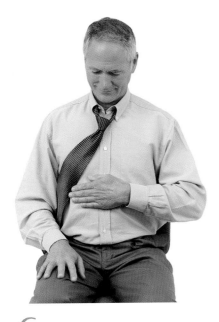

6 Complete the sequence by gently stroking your abdomen with the flat of your left hand working in a clockwise direction to help calm and soothe the area.

TOP TIPS

◆ Eat small meals at regular intervals. Always sit down to eat, allow plenty of time, and chew your food well. Do not rush. Aim to finish your last main meal at least 2 hours before going to bed.

◆ If you often suffer from indigestion, cut back on spicy, foods, strong coffee, alcohol, tobacco, or fizzy drinks, as these can cause heartburn.

◆ Sipping chamomile, fennel, or peppermint tea after meals can aid digestion and help prevent heartburn.

WARNING

Avoid this massage if you are pregnant or have your period, unless advised otherwise by your physician.

Long-haul DVT (DEEP VEIN THROMBOSIS)

The formation of blood clots in the deep veins—known as deep vein thrombosis (DVT)—is often a concern on long airplane flights. But sitting still in any confined space —whether at home, at work, or in a bus, train or automobile —can also slow blood flow in the legs and feet, increasing the risk of DVT.

Use this 5-minute routine to improve the flow of blood back to your heart. Practice this exercise wherever you are to maintain healthy circulation in legs and feet.

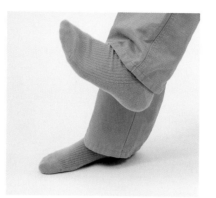
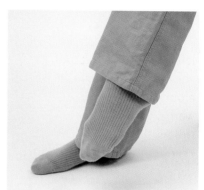

1 Raise one foot a little way off the floor. Trace a circle with your raised foot in a counterclockwise direction. Make 5 circles. Repeat in other direction. Repeat with other foot.

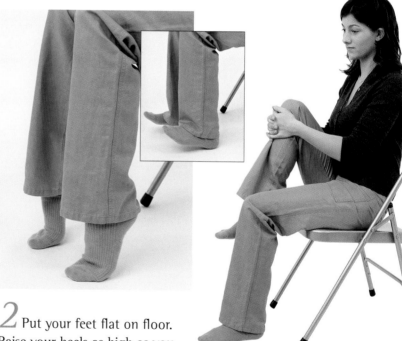

2 Put your feet flat on floor. Raise your heels as high as you can, with the balls of your feet on the floor. Put your feet down. Repeat 2 or 3 times. Point your toes up, keeping heels still. Put them down. Repeat 2 or 3 times.

3 Now raise your right leg and bend your knee toward your chest. Keep your body straight and hold for a count of 5. Slowly return your foot to the floor. Repeat 4 or 5 times with each leg.

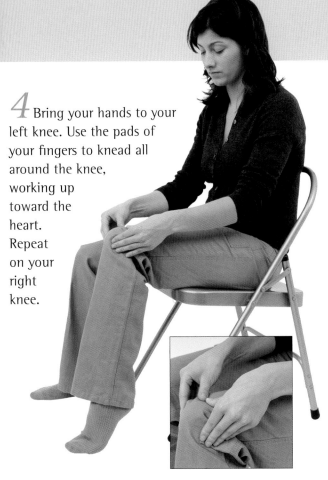

4 Bring your hands to your left knee. Use the pads of your fingers to knead all around the knee, working up toward the heart. Repeat on your right knee.

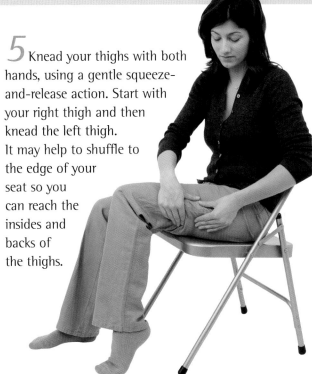

5 Knead your thighs with both hands, using a gentle squeeze-and-release action. Start with your right thigh and then knead the left thigh. It may help to shuffle to the edge of your seat so you can reach the insides and backs of the thighs.

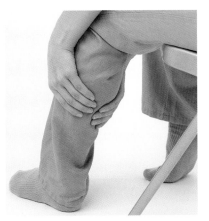

6 Place your hands on either side of the left calf. Gently rock your hands from side to side, working from ankle to the back of the knee. Feel the muscle wobble under your touch. Keep hands soft and relaxed with light pressure. Repeat on the right calf.

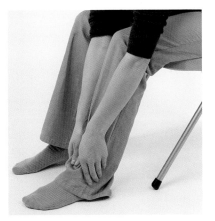

7 Finish with deep stroking, both hands together. Begin with the right leg. Clasp your hands around the ankle, slide them up the calf and around knee and thigh. Use firm but comfortable pressure on the upward stroke. Repeat 3 times on both legs.

TOP TIPS

◆ Wear loose clothing and avoid socks with tight elastic below the knees—a red ring around your leg is a telltale sign that they are too tight.

◆ Have a medical exam before flying if you suffer from varicose veins, have a history of cardiovascular problems, are pregnant, overweight, or have any concerns about your health. Your physician may recommend the use of support stockings or suggest you take an aspirin to thin your blood just before flying.

Jet lag: DAYTIME ARRIVAL

Crossing time zones can upset the body's biological clock and cause disturbed sleep patterns, tiredness, and irregular appetite commonly known as jet lag. Eastward journeys tend to be worse than westward flights. It's hard to eliminate jet lag totally, but you can minimize the effects.

Here are two quick self-massage sequences. The first is for daytime arrivals, to help you stay awake; the second is for nighttime arrivals, when you need to try to sleep, even though you may not feel tired.

If you arrive during the day, try to stay awake and go to bed at the local time. Use this reviving massage routine to help your body clock readjust. If possible, do the massage outdoors and follow it with a gentle walk in the fresh air. The exercise stimulates the blood circulation, while exposure to sunlight helps reduce the body's levels of the sleep-inducing hormone melatonin. You can do the massage standing or sitting.

TOP TIPS

◆ Aim to get plenty of sleep before you travel so that your body is rested and more able to adapt to the time changes.

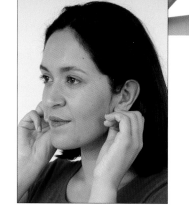

1 Massaging your ears can stimulate and revitalize your whole body. Gently knead and squeeze your ears between thumbs and first fingers. Begin at the tops of your ears and work down to your lobes. When you reach the lobes, give a gentle tug. Repeat 3 times.

2 Cover your ears with your palms. Gently circle the heels of your hands in whichever direction feels best for you. Start slowly, and gradually speed up. Enjoy the tingling sensation this brings. Continue for 30 seconds.

TECHNIQUE CHECKLIST

◆ Kneading ◆ Stretching ◆ Pressures (see pages 38–55)

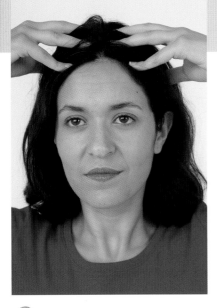

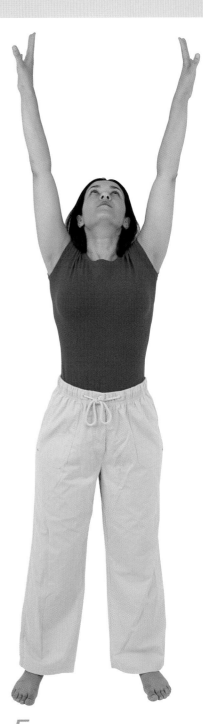

3 Place your hands in clawlike position on top of your head. With fingertips "glued" to scalp, gently vibrate your hands. Move to another position on your head and repeat. Cover the whole head.

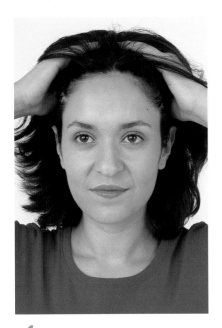

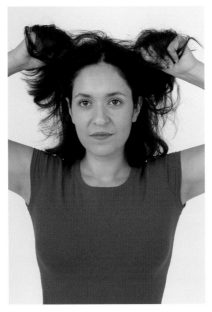

4 Draw your hands through your hair and allow them to rest on your head with palms facing downward. Now bring your fingers together to clasp a handful of hair in each loose fist. Give it a gentle twist and then a light tug. Release. Move your hands to clasp another section of hair. Repeat until you have covered the whole scalp.

5 Finish with a full body stretch. Place your arms above your head and inhale as you stretch a little backward. Breathe out as you relax the stretch. Repeat 3 times.

Jet lag: NIGHTTIME ARRIVAL

The secret of minimizing jet lag when you arrive in the dark is to go to bed at the local time, even though you may not be feeling tired. However, it can be difficult enough trying to relax when you are staying in a strange hotel room away from your usual home comforts, without the effect on your body clock of switching time zones.

To help you relax and induce sleepy feelings, fill a bathtub with warm, soapy water as soon as you get to your destination. Add 5 drops of lavender essential oil to the water to enhance the sleep-inducing effects. Then have a long, relaxing soak.

Dress in comfy night clothes and follow this 5-minute sequence to calm your mind and body and help you get to sleep. The massage begins with your feet; relaxing the sensory nerve endings here can have a wonderfully soothing effect on the whole body. You can do these movements while sitting on a chair or on the side of the bed.

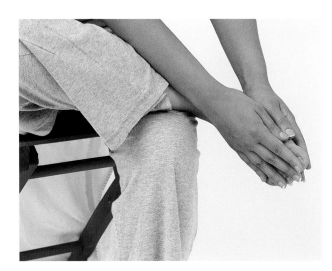

1 Rest one foot on your other leg and cradle it in the palms of your hands. Hold for a few minutes. Feel the warmth of your hands helping your foot to relax. Concentrate on slowing down your breathing. Gently stroke the foot with one or both hands moving together.

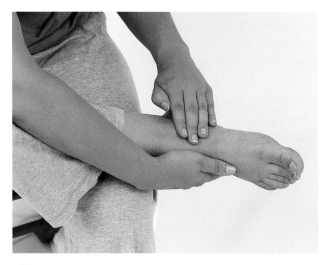

2 Using the flats of your fingers and palms, gently stroke around the whole foot and ankle. Try slow circular stroking or longer strokes, whichever you find the most soothing. Keep going as long as you wish. Now change feet.

TECHNIQUE CHECKLIST

◆ Acupressure   ◆ Pressures   ◆ Kneading   ◆ Stroking   ◆ Feathering   ◆ Stretching   (see pages 38–55)

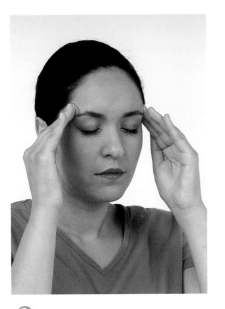

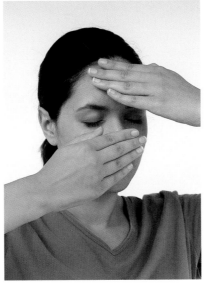

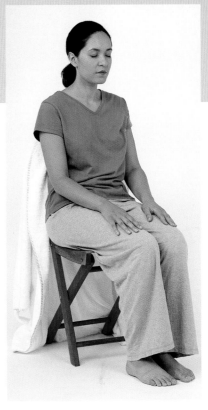

3 Bring your hands to your temples. Close your eyes. Use the pads of first and second fingers to make slow circular rotations. Feel the skin moving. Repeat the words "slow and gentle" to yourself to help you calm your movements.

4 Relax the muscles in your forehead with some gentle stroking (see pages 42-43). Keep your eyes closed and stroke from brows to hairline with your hands working alternately. Continue for as long as you wish.

5 Finish by sitting comfortably with your hands resting on your thighs. Enjoy the stillness this brings. Try to switch off from any outside noise and concentrate on listening to the gentle ebb and flow of your breathing.

Acupressure for blocked ears

If your ears are blocked or ringing after a long flight, use the acupoint in front of the middle of your ear to clear them. To locate the point, open your mouth and feel for the slight hollow there. Apply pressure with your first or second fingers. Hold for 30 seconds and release.

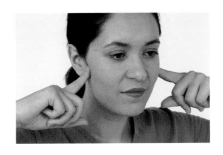

Acupressure for motion sickness

To combat the nausea caused by movement, locate the acupressure point on the inside of your arm, about 3 fingers' width above the natural crease on your wrist. Support your lower arm with your fingers and apply pressure with the pad of your thumb. Hold for 30 seconds and release. Change to the other arm. Repeat as necessary.

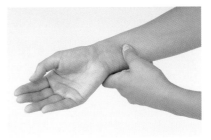

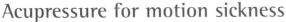

Shopping-bag strain

Carrying heavy bags can put a great strain on the muscles in your hands, arms, and shoulders—not to mention your back! Use some or all of the steps in this 10-minute self-massage sequence to warm up before and after your trip—when you stop for a coffee or whenever you feel tingling or aches and pains. The steps can easily be performed while standing or sitting.

TOP TIPS

◆ Balance your load. Never carry a heavy bag in one hand or on one shoulder. Divide the contents between two bags to ensure your back, shoulders, and arms all take a share of the weight.

1 Begin by relaxing your shoulders. Push one shoulder slightly forward and the other a little way back. Now roll your shoulders backward in a flowing, circular rhythm. One shoulder moves after the other. Continue for 30 seconds.

2 Hold both hands up above your head. Now stretch up with your left arm, then with your right arm. Repeat 10 times.

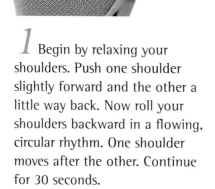

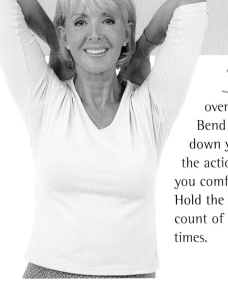

3 Bring both arms over and behind your head. Bend your elbows, and reach down your back. Do not force the action; only reach as far as you comfortably can. Hold the stretch for a count of 5. Repeat 3 times.

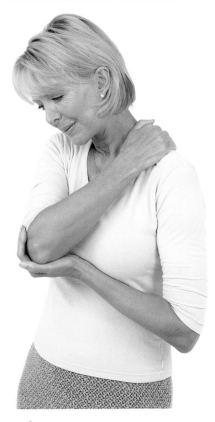

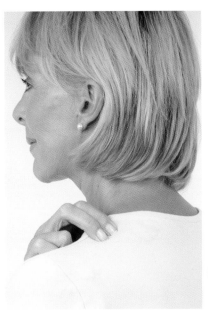

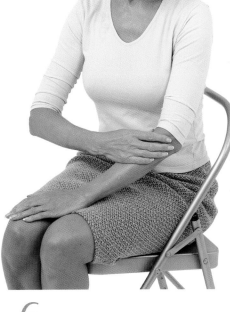

4 Place your right hand on your left shoulder, fingers pointing down your back. Support your right elbow in your left hand. Feel for the fleshy muscle across the top of the shoulder, and grasp it between fingers and thumb. Hold and gently squeeze for a count of 5. Work backward and forward along your shoulder using this clasp-squeeze-hold-and-release movement. Repeat on the other side.

5 With your hands still in the same position, gently press two fingertips into the fleshy area along the top of your shoulder. Apply pressure on one spot and then slowly rotate the fingertips. Lift your fingers and move to an adjacent trouble spot. Repeat until you have covered the whole area. Repeat along the muscle at the top of the other shoulder. This muscle stores much tension, causing stiff neck and shoulders.

6 The next four steps help release tension in the forearms. Start by stroking up your forearm from fingers to elbow, using the flat of your other hand and maintaining a firm but comfortable pressure. Keep your hand relaxed and molded to the contours of your arms. When you reach the elbow, glide lightly back to the fingers and repeat. Continue as long as you wish. Repeat on the other arm. ➤

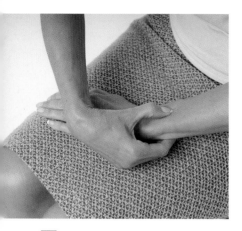

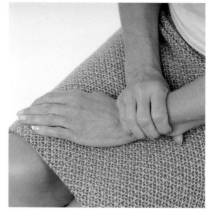

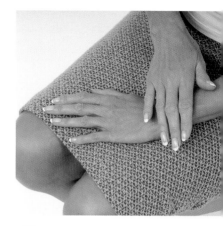

7 Grasp your forearm in the V between the thumb and first finger of your other hand, thumb on top and fingers beneath. Use your thumb to make gentle static pressures up the center of your outer forearm, beginning just above the wrist. Press, hold for a count of 3, and then release. Move to the next spot and repeat. Continue to your elbow. Repeat on the other arm.

8 Grip and squeeze your wrist. Hold for a count of 5. Repeat 3 times on each wrist, placing your working hand in a slightly different position on the wrist each time.

9 Cover your outer wrist with gentle, soothing strokes, using the flat of your hand. Repeat these comforting strokes on the inside of your wrist.

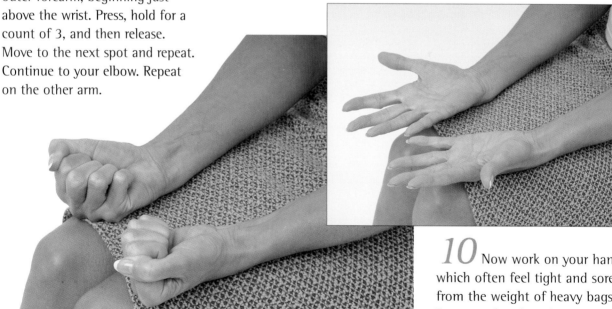

10 Now work on your hands, which often feel tight and sore from the weight of heavy bags. Rest your hands, palms upward, in front of you. Clench your fists and hold for a count of 5. Release and stretch your fingers and thumbs out as far as you can. Hold for the count of 5. Release and repeat 3 times.

TECHNIQUE CHECKLIST

◆ Stretching ◆ Kneading ◆ Stroking ◆ Holding (see pages 38–55)

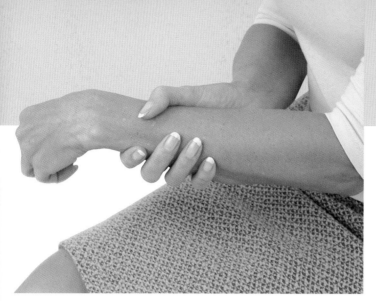

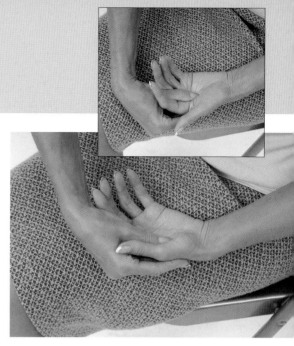

11 Support your left wrist by clasping your lower arm firmly with your right hand. Now make a soft fist with your left hand and gently rotate the wrist in a clockwise direction. Keep your supporting hand still. Make 3 rotations; then change direction and repeat. Repeat with your right wrist.

12 With the left palm upward, use the thumb and first finger of the right hand to grasp the webbing between thumb and first finger of the left hand. With thumb on top, squeeze and hold for a count of 5. Repeat all around the muscular pad at the base of the thumb and between the fingers. Repeat on the other hand.

TOP TIPS

◆ When carrying heavy goods, use a backpack with two straps whenever possible. This leaves your hands free to carry lighter bags.

13 Turn your hand over and offer a soothing touch to your whole arm with some firm stroking from your fingers to your shoulders.

14 Complete the sequence by shaking away any remaining tension. With your arms held in front of you, keep your wrists relaxed and enjoy the freedom of a loose, shaking movement. Do around 5 shakes.

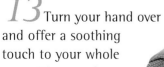

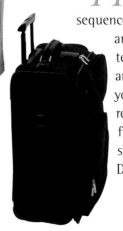

Poor posture

Standing or sitting with poor posture creates tension in the back, neck, and shoulders, and can lead to stiffness, headache, poor circulation, shallow breathing, and even eyestrain. Good posture boosts health and vitality, often contributing to greater self-confidence.

This sequence helps you work through your body to check your posture. You may find it helpful to stand in front of a mirror. Begin at your feet and move upward, finishing with your head.

TECHNIQUE CHECKLIST

◆ Stretching   ◆ Kneading   (see pages 38–55)

2 Bring your hands to your knees and gently knead around the kneecap to release any tension. Bring your upper body back to standing position with knees relaxed, (neither rigid, nor bent). Allow your weight to drop through your heels.

1 Stand with your feet about 12 in. (30 cm) apart, and parallel. Lift and spread your toes so that you have a solid base to stand on. Rock backward and forward twice. Now sway from one foot to the other. Check that your weight is evenly distributed on your feet.

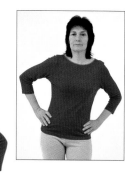

3 Make 5 circular movements with your pelvis moving in one direction. Repeat in the other direction. This will release any tension in your lower back. Now tilt your pelvis forward and backward. Find a balance at midpoint. This helps keep the back in its natural position, neither arching nor slumping.

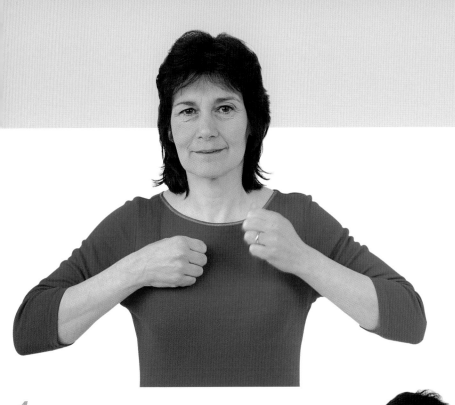

4 Turn your attention to the chest. Make soft fists with your hands and gently beat your chest, using the flats of your fingers and the heels of your hands—not your knuckles. Now lift your rib cage upward to open your chest and encourage deeper breathing.

5 Bring your shoulders up toward your ears. Hold for a count of 3. Release. Repeat. Pull your shoulders down and away from your ears so they are relaxed, not slouching forward or pulled backward. Check that your shoulders are at the same height. Allow your arms to hang loosely by your sides.

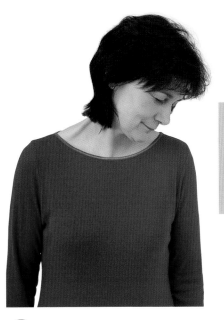

WARNING
Do not rotate your head to the back, since this can lead to neck injury.

6 Drop your head gently to one side, then to the front, and across your chest to the other side. Repeat. Lengthen your neck so that your head is balanced evenly and freely on top of your spine. Your chin should be neither tucked in nor protruding forward.

7 Imagine there is an invisible cord running from the top of your head to the ceiling, giving you a tall, relaxed posture. Try to stay in this position for several minutes. Is it difficult? Does it feel unnatural? If so, this is an early indication that you are starting to develop poor postural habits.

Practice this sequence regularly to correct them.

Cramps

Cramps are a result of sudden contraction of a muscle, often causing extreme pain. Cramps often hit when you least expect them. You may find that you get cramps at night, during or after exercise, or when you have been sitting still for a long time.

There can be many causes, including poor circulation, repetitive actions, and sitting or lying in an awkward position. One of the best ways to alleviate cramps is to gently stretch the affected muscle and then ease it with massage.

Cramping in your legs

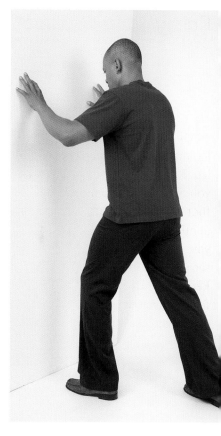

1 Begin by facing a wall. Stand about 20 in. (50 cm) away from the wall and place your hands against it. Put the cramped leg behind you as far as you comfortably can. Keep both feet flat on the ground. Now bend your front knee and slowly lean forward against the wall, without allowing your back foot to rise from the ground. Feel the stretch in your calf muscle and the gradual release of the cramping sensation. Hold for a count of at least 10. Repeat if you wish.

2 Knead your calf muscle using one or both hands. Do this with a leg resting on a chair or sitting with your legs outstretched, with the cramped leg on top of the other. Squeeze, roll, and release the muscle between your fingers and the heel of your hand using firm pressure. Finish by stroking from your ankles to your knees to soothe the area and encourage the flow of blood back to the heart.

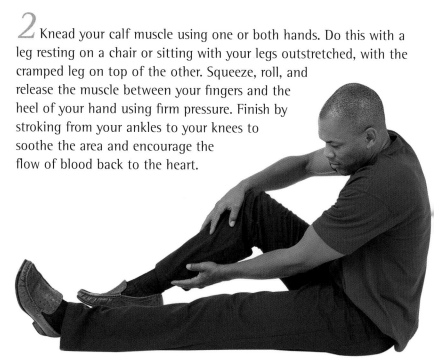

Cramping in your feet

1 Sit on the floor or your bed with your affected leg outstretched and resting on top of your other leg. Now stretch your toes toward you. If you are able to reach your foot with your hands, gently pull it toward you. Hold for 10 seconds and release. Repeat until you feel the cramps subsiding.

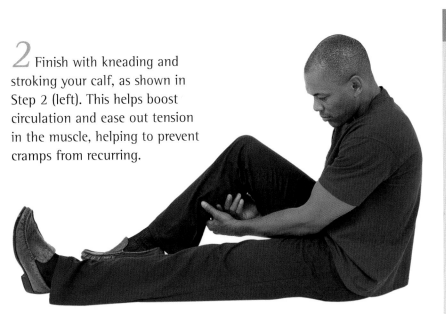

2 Finish with kneading and stroking your calf, as shown in Step 2 (left). This helps boost circulation and ease out tension in the muscle, helping to prevent cramps from recurring.

TECHNIQUE CHECKLIST

◆ Stretching   ◆ Kneading   ◆ Stroking (see pages 38–55)

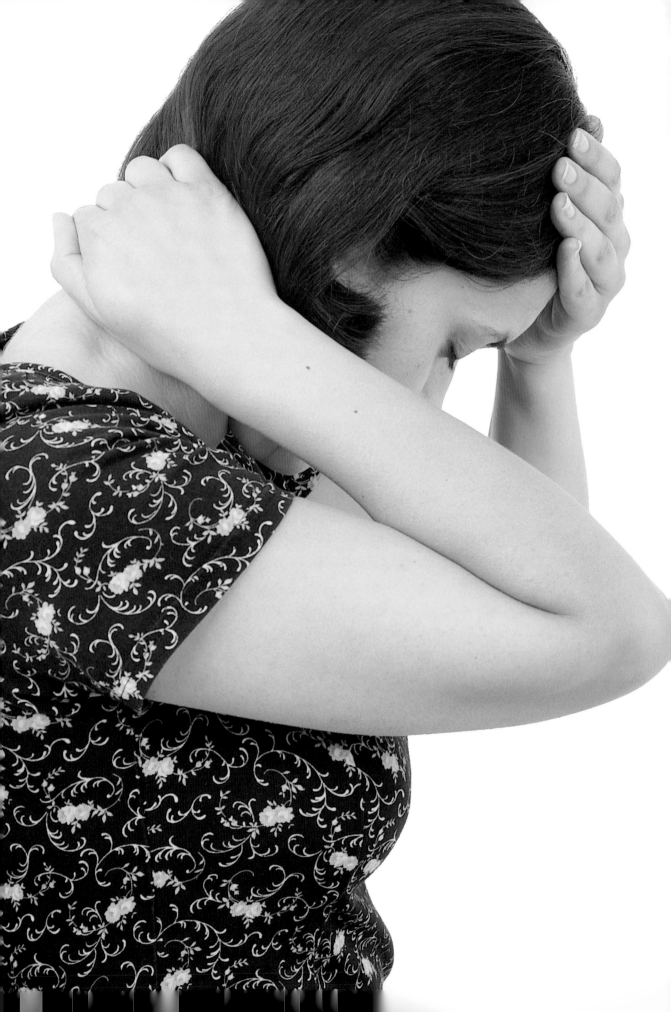

6 AT WORK

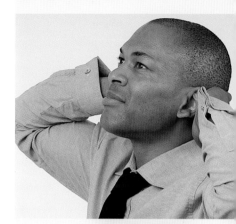

Whether you are working in a busy office or on your own, there are bound to be days when you feel tired, stressed, and irritable. Many employers are encouraging self-massage in the workplace because it has been shown to help improve mental alertness, performance, and productivity and reduce the number of "sick" days due to stress. However tight your deadlines, it is worthwhile setting aside 10 minutes each day to perform one of the following self-massage sequences.

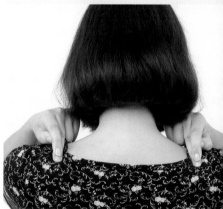

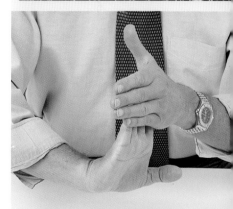

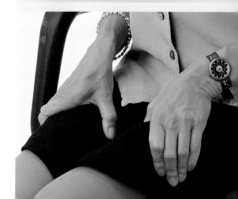

Tension headache

Tension headache is often triggered by poor posture or stress factors such as working under pressure. When you notice the first signs of a headache, a head-and-shoulder massage can often ease away the tension in taut muscles and restore healthy circulation to the area, lifting or reducing the pain.

The pressure should be firm enough to be effective without making a headache worse. Keep the movements slow and controlled. If possible, try to find a quiet place away from any noise. Dim the lighting, and let fresh air circulate around the room.

1 Try to ease yourself into relaxation. Close your eyes. Cradle your head securely in your hands, fingers meeting on the top of your head. As you breathe out, exert a gentle pressure with your hands. As you breathe in, release the pressure. Move your hands a little farther back and repeat.

WARNING

Most headaches are not a cause for concern. However, you should seek medical advice if the pain is persistent or very severe, or if it is accompanied by fever, vomiting, altered vision, a stiff neck, or a rash.

2 Lean your head sideways toward your left shoulder. Place your left hand on top of your head. Gently clasp your head. Allow your hand to rest on your head without pulling. Hold for a count of 5, then release. Bring your arms to your sides and repeat on the other side. Do not force this movement. Stop if you feel any discomfort. To enhance the benefits of the stretch, concentrate on your breathing.

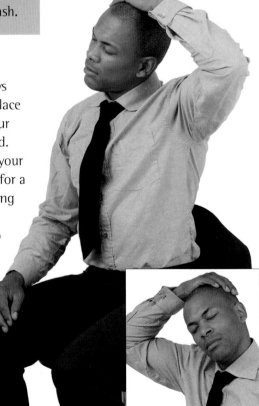

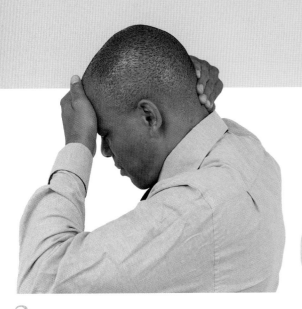

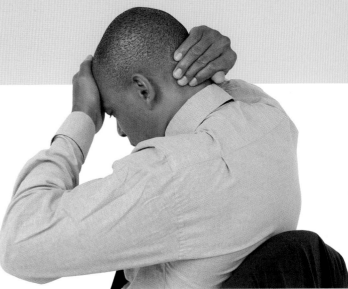

3 Tilt your head forward a little. Place one hand on your forehead for support, and use the palm of your other hand to stroke the back of your neck gently in a large circular movement. Repeat several times.

4 With your hands held in the same position, lightly squeeze and roll the muscles at the back of your neck between your thumb and the flats of all 4 fingers. Repeat using the other hand.

TOP TIPS

◆ Among the acupressure points that ease headaches is one at the center of your forehead, just above the bridge of your nose and halfway between the inner end of your eyebrows. Locate the point with your first or second finger. Press and hold for 5–10 seconds. Release and repeat.

5 Still supporting your forehead with one hand, gently rub up the back of your neck and along the bony ridge at the base of your skull to your ears. Use the flats of your fingers or the sides of your hands—whichever feels best for you.   →

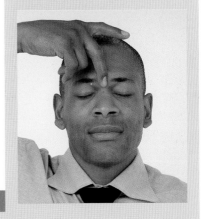

TECHNIQUE CHECKLIST

◆ Kneading   ◆ Stroking   ◆ Feathering   ◆ Rubbing   ◆ Pressures   ◆ Holding (see pages 38–55)

Tension headache...continued

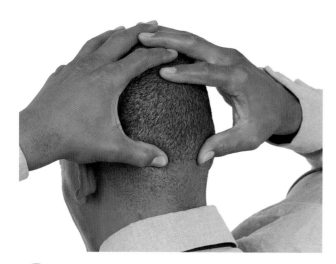

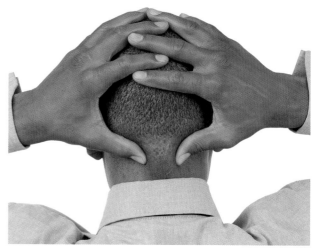

6 Now place both hands on your head with your thumbs resting on the bony ridge. Locate the slight hollows at the base of the skull on either side of your neck, and rest your thumbs on this acupoint. Gently tilt your head back a little way so the weight of your head on your thumbs increases the pressure. Hold for 20–30 seconds. Release and repeat.

7 Now make small pressures with the pads of your thumbs along the ridge, working from the center toward your ears. Begin with a fairly light pressure and gradually increase the depth to suit your own comfort. Return to the starting point and repeat 3 times.

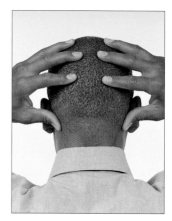

8 Place one hand on top of your head. With the flat of your hand molded to the shape of your head, gently knead your scalp between your fingers and the heel of your hand. Feel your scalp relaxing as you massage away the tension. Repeat with the other hand.

TOP TIPS

◆ Lavender essential oil is a widely used remedy for tension headaches. Whenever a headache strikes, simply apply 2 drops to a tissue and inhale, or place 1 drop on the first fingers of both hands and gently massage your temples.

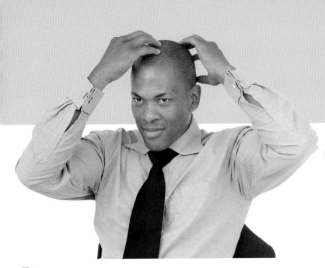

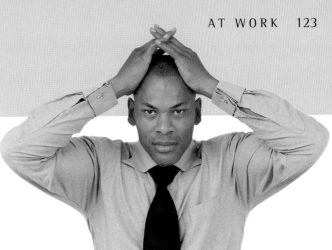

9 Now rake through your scalp with the tips of your fingers. Start at your hairline and rake back firmly along the scalp, down to the base of the skull. Cover the whole scalp. Your hands can work at the same time or with an alternate raking action.

10 Interlock your fingers on top of your head. Slowly press the heels of your hands inward and upward against the side of your head. Feel your scalp moving beneath your touch. Move to another position and repeat.

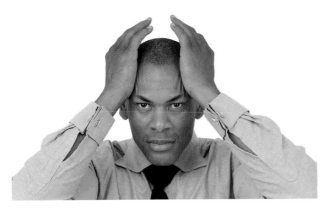

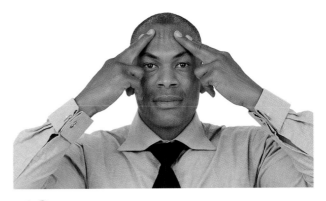

11 Lower your hands a little so that the heels of your hands are resting on your temples. Make at least 10 circular movements with the heels of your hands, clockwise or counterclockwise, whichever suits you best. Keep the movement very slow.

12 Glide your hands up to your forehead and use the pads of your first and second fingers to make small rotations, working from the center to your temples. Repeat these gentle circular movements all over your forehead, including your eyebrows.

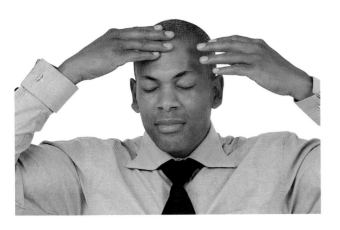

13 Finish with slow, nurturing strokes across your forehead. Use the pads of the fingertips of both hands to stroke gently from the center to your ears. Keep the pressure light and nurturing. Stroke for as long as you wish.

Lack of focus

If you find it hard to stay focused and spend too long with your "head in the clouds," this 5-minute routine will help you focus your thoughts and bring you back down to earth. This routine can also help you remain calm before a nerve-racking event, such as an interview.

The exercise is performed here while standing, but it can easily be adapted for sitting in a chair if you prefer.

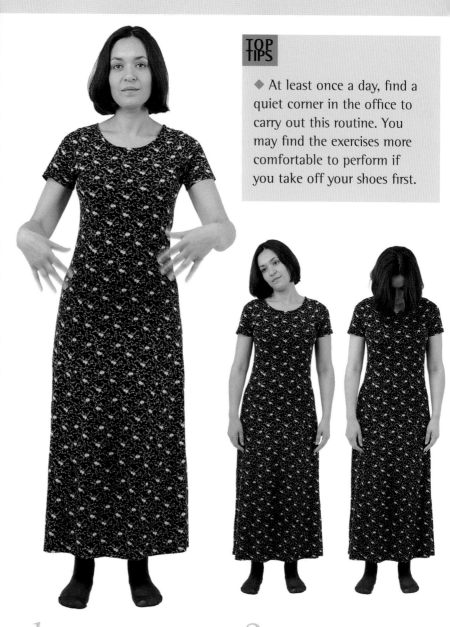

TOP TIPS

◆ At least once a day, find a quiet corner in the office to carry out this routine. You may find the exercises more comfortable to perform if you take off your shoes first.

1 Start by shaking your hands to release any tension. Hold your hands in front of you and shake them loosely from your wrist for a count of 10.

2 Gently circle your head to loosen your neck. Drop your head to your right side toward one shoulder then circle it forward and to your left shoulder. Trace this arc in the opposite direction, circling your head forward and to your right shoulder, keeping the movement slow and controlled. Repeat.

TECHNIQUE CHECKLIST

◆ Stretching   ◆ Stroking (see pages 38–55)

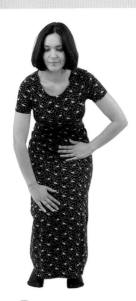
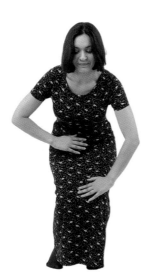
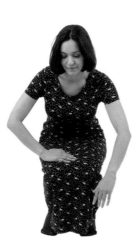
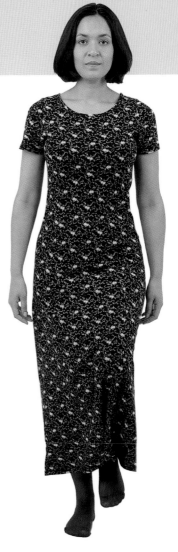

3 Still in a standing position, brush yourself down with the flats of your hands, using long sweeping strokes. Work from your head to your toes, bending your knees to reach your calves. When you reach your feet, give your hands a shake to help release any negativity, and then repeat the downward strokes.

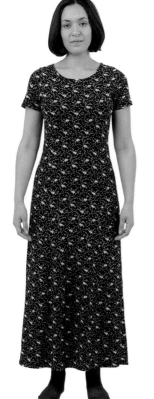

TOP TIPS

◆ Find a simple strategy to use when your thoughts start to wander. Try a verbal cue, such as "stop," or make your hands into fists and then release them.

4 Focus your attention on your feet. Wiggle your toes and gently stamp your feet on the floor. Feel the solid ground beneath you, supporting you.

5 Now stand still in a relaxed position with your feet firmly on the ground, shoulder-width apart. Let your knees relax a little, and hang your arms loosely by your sides. Relax your shoulders. Keep your eyes open and look ahead. Breathe normally. In this position, imagine your feet are like the roots of a tree, growing deep into the earth. Your body is stable, like the trunk of a tree. Try to connect with the powerful strength of the earth beneath your feet. This is a practice known as "grounding," and it is used to help you concentrate on the "here and now." Stand in this position for a few minutes, enjoying the inner quietness of mind and body. Now repeat Steps 1 and 2.

Eyestrain

Working at a computer screen or watching television can put a strain on the muscles in the eyes because they are working hard to maintain focus. This can often lead to blurred vision and headaches. The next time your eyes feel tired, try this 5-minute massage routine. You may rest your elbows on a table or desk if this makes it more comfortable.

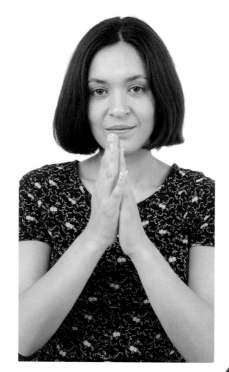

1 Rub your hands together so they feel warm.

2 Now cup the palms of your hands over your eyes. Close your fingers to shut out as much light as possible. Enjoy the restful warmth and darkness for a couple of minutes—or longer if you have time. This technique is known as palming.

TOP TIPS

◆ To avoid eyestrain, blink frequently throughout the day. It's estimated that we should blink about 15 times a minute.

◆ Ensure you have good light when reading, writing, or working at a computer. Ideally, the light should come from over your left shoulder if you are right-handed, and over your right shoulder if you are left-handed.

TECHNIQUE CHECKLIST

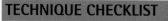

◆ Rubbing ◆ Holding ◆ Stroking ◆ Pressures ◆ Tapping (see pages 38–55)

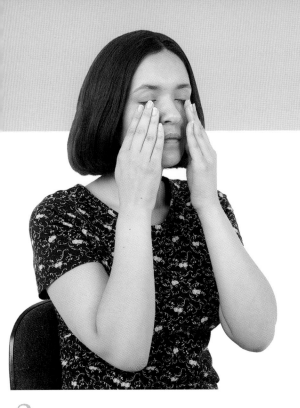

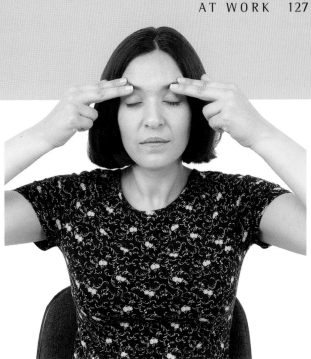

3 Draw your hands across your cheeks toward your ears in a gentle smoothing action to help boost blood circulation to the area. Repeat 6 times.

4 Place the tips of your first and second fingers just above the inner ends of your eyebrows. Apply static pressures along the eyebrow to the outer edge. Press, hold, and release. Continue along the bone beneath your eyes (avoiding the delicate skin around your eyes), working outward. When you reach the outer edge, return to the starting point. Repeat 3 times. Now stroke over your eyebrows.

TOP TIPS

◆ Helpful acupoints are located in the hollows level with the outside corners of the eyes (see page 53). Apply pressure with the first or second finger, angled away from the eye. Hold for 5–10 seconds. Release and repeat. Use to relieve tired eyes and headaches and to clear your vision, especially after long periods working at a computer screen.

◆ If you suffer from tired eyes, try palming for 10 minutes 2 or 3 times a day. Listen to soothing music at the same time to help you relax.

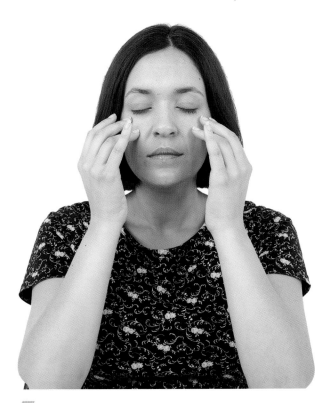

5 Next tap around your eye area using the pads of the fingers of both hands. Maintain a gentle pressure and avoid working directly over your eyes.

6 Finish by blinking your eyes tightly several times. Open your eyes and look into the distance. Try to take regular breaks and look out the window.

Concentration dips

We all have "dips" in concentration at one time or another during the workday. You may find that your attention starts to wander just before or just after lunch, for example. Try this sequence to restore mental alertness and help you stay sharp. The whole routine takes less than 5 minutes but can make a big difference to your concentration level.

1 Make loose fists with both hands and gently beat all over your head using a drumming action. Make sure you use the flats of your fingers and heels of your hands—not the knuckles.

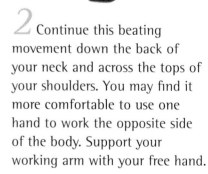

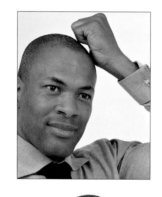

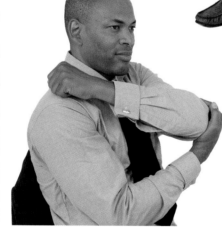

2 Continue this beating movement down the back of your neck and across the tops of your shoulders. You may find it more comfortable to use one hand to work the opposite side of the body. Support your working arm with your free hand.

3 Starting from the same position as the previous move, rub across your shoulders with the flat of your hand. Use a light, brisk rubbing action as far as you can reach across your upper back, up your neck, and over your chest. Repeat on the other side.

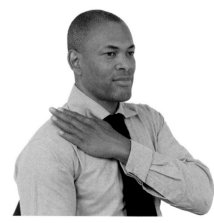

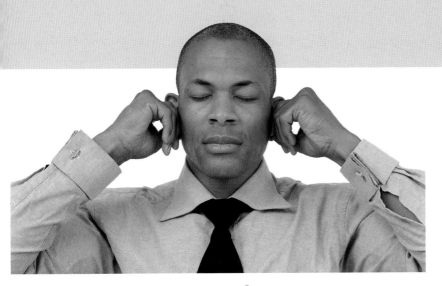

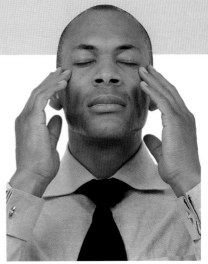

◆ The brain is 80 percent water. Drink plenty of water to help improve mental agility and maintain concentration levels.

4 Move your hands to your ears and gently rotate them forward and then backward. Now place your hands on your forehead and gently rake them up and down, working from the center outward.

5 Close your eyes and lightly tap all over your face with the pads of your fingertips.

◆ Take regular meals to stabilize your blood-sugar levels. Brain cells need energy to function properly, and skipping meals can diminish your powers of concentration.

◆The color yellow is linked with wisdom. Surround yourself with yellow to help focus your attention and stimulate your mind.

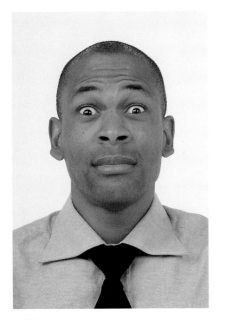

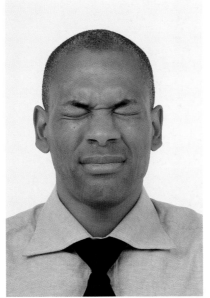

6 When you have covered your whole face, raise your eyebrows and open your eyes wide. Finally, blink several times.

TECHNIQUE CHECKLIST

◆ Beating   ◆ Rubbing   ◆ Tapping   ◆ Stroking   (see pages 38–55)

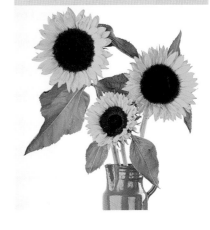

Fatigue

When your energy levels are low, try this simple massage sequence. It takes only 5–10 minutes but can invigorate both mind and body, providing an instant pick-me-up when you need it.

Kick off your shoes and use these stimulating moves to wake yourself up, clear your head, and increase your energy levels at any time during a busy workday.

1 With your arms down by your sides, raise one shoulder up as the other goes down. Repeat in a rapid action about 20 times.

2 Sitting in a chair, turn from your waist as far as you can to look back over one shoulder. Hold for a count of 6. Now look back over the other shoulder. Repeat the movements.

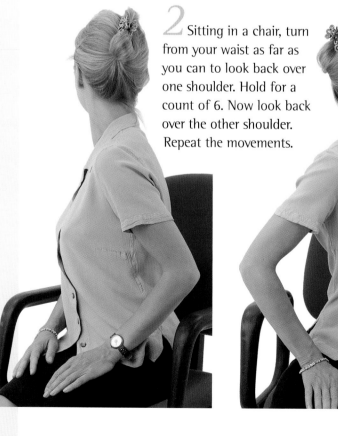

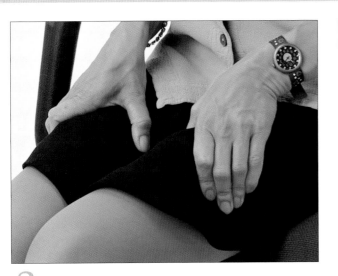

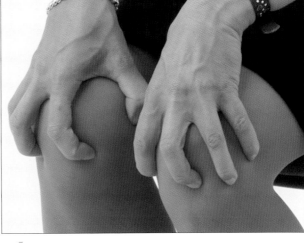

3 Place the palms of your hands on your thighs. Use your fingers and thumbs to produce a slight squeezing action over the muscles in the tops of your legs, working from your hips down to your knees. Repeat several times. Finish with a brisk sweeping motion in the same direction.

4 Holding your knees in the palms of your hands, gently massage them with your fingers, using small circular movements. Work all around the kneecaps.

5 Place your hands on top of your head and use your fingertips to gently tap the scalp. Imagine you are playing the piano. Cover your whole head with this tapping action to stimulate your brain. Continue over the forehead, temples, cheeks, and neck. ➡

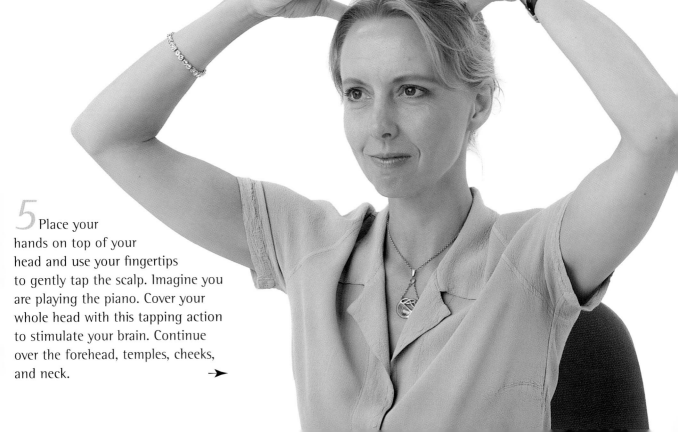

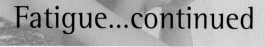

Fatigue...continued

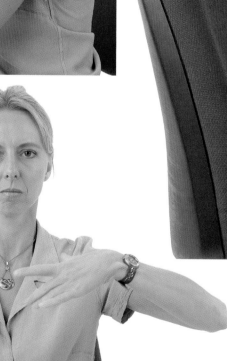

6 Make a loose fist with one hand and use the flat edge of your knuckles to gently beat the shoulders and upper back on the opposite side of your body. Use your other hand to support the elbow of the working arm. Feel your body begin to tingle.

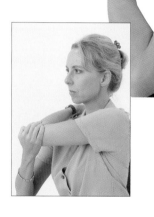

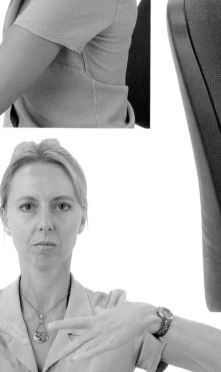

7 Place your arms by your sides. Keeping your arms loose and relaxed, shake your hands vigorously. Repeat with your arms held at chest height, and then above your head.

TOP TIPS

◆ Dehydration can leave you feeling lethargic. Keep a bottle of water at home, at work, and in the car, and replenish your fluid levels throughout the day.

8 Interlock your fingers and stretch your arms out in front of you at shoulder height. Turn your palms to face forward with your thumbs down. Gently push the heels of your hands forward so that you feel an energizing stretch from wrist to fingertips. Hold for a count of 5. Release and repeat.

TOP TIPS

◆ For an instant zing, place a couple of drops of rosemary pure essential oil on a tissue and inhale the aroma. Rosemary stimulates the nervous system, lifts mental fatigue, improves memory, alertness, and concentration, and eases aches and pains.

TOP TIPS

◆ Whenever you get the chance, run up and down the stairs to boost your energy levels throughout the day.

9 Sitting with bent knees, lift one heel off the floor, followed by the other, as if running on the spot. Continue for about 1 minute.

10 Finish by moving your neck slowly from side to side and then in gentle forward semicircles. Do not force the movement.

TECHNIQUE CHECKLIST

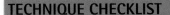

◆ Stretching ◆ Kneading ◆ Tapping ◆ Beating (see pages 38–55)

Repetitive strain injury (RSI)

Many jobs today involve continuous, repetitive hand movements. Over time, these frequent movements can lead to inflammation of the delicate tendons in the hands, leading to numbness and pain—a condition called repetitive strain injury (RSI). To prevent RSI, it is vital to correct your posture.

Regular gentle stretching and massage can also help avoid or alleviate RSI. Do this short stretch and massage routine at regular times throughout the day. Stop or limit the movement if you experience pain or discomfort.

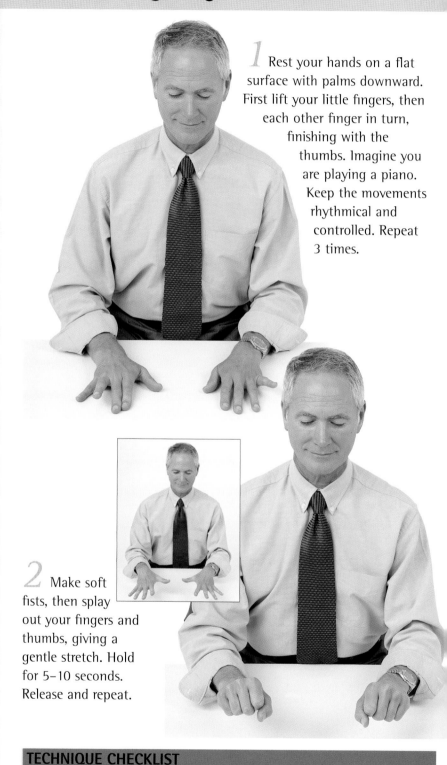

1 Rest your hands on a flat surface with palms downward. First lift your little fingers, then each other finger in turn, finishing with the thumbs. Imagine you are playing a piano. Keep the movements rhythmical and controlled. Repeat 3 times.

2 Make soft fists, then splay out your fingers and thumbs, giving a gentle stretch. Hold for 5–10 seconds. Release and repeat.

TECHNIQUE CHECKLIST

◆ Stretching   ◆ Kneading   ◆ Pressures   ◆ Stroking   (see pages 38–55)

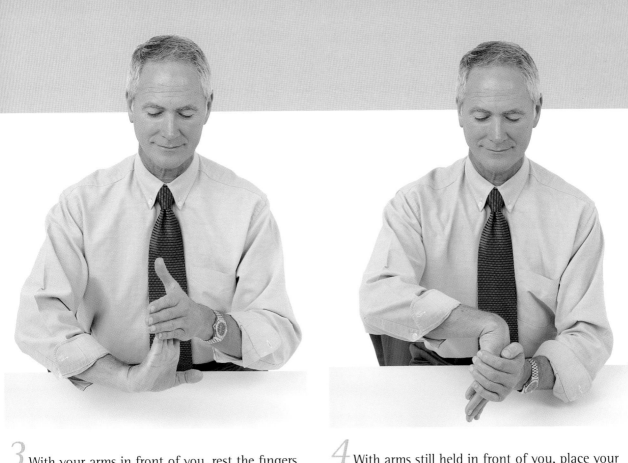

3 With your arms in front of you, rest the fingers of your right hand in your left palm. Bend the right hand at the wrist and gently press the fingers with your left hand until you feel a gentle stretch in your right wrist. Stop if this causes discomfort. Hold for 10 seconds. Release and repeat on the other hand.

4 With arms still held in front of you, place your left hand on top of your right hand and gently press it down so the right wrist is stretched in the opposite direction to that of the previous move. Release and repeat on the other hand.

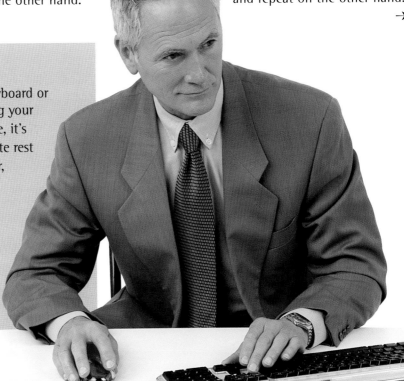

TOP TIPS

◆ Take regular breaks from the keyboard or from other repetitive work involving your hands and fingers. As a general rule, it's a good idea to take a 1-to-2-minute rest every 15–20 minutes, with a longer, 5-to-10 minute break every hour.

◆ Take time to adjust your work posture and workstation to minimize the physical stress involved in using a keyboard. It really is worth making the effort for the sake of your long-term health.

Repetitive strain injury...continued

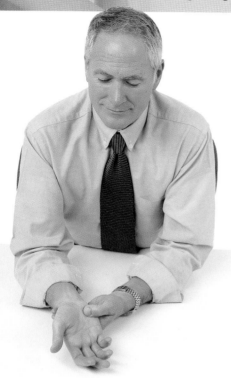

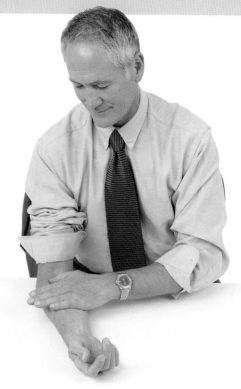

5 Clasp your right hand in your left hand, and use your left thumb to gently knead your right palm with small circular rotations. Work all over the palm, between the fingers, and along the fingers. Include the heel of the hand. Feel any areas of tension and gently ease these through massage. Continue these circular kneading strokes from wrist to elbow.

6 Use the flat of your hand to make circular rotations up your inner forearm, working from the wrist to the elbow crease. Keep the movement fairly brisk and stimulating to encourage blood circulation to the area. Turn your arm over and repeat on your outer forearm.

TOP TIPS

◆ Cradling the phone between your ear and shoulder can cause serious long-term neck and shoulder problems. If your job involves simultaneously talking on the phone and using a computer keyboard or writing notes, use a telephone with a headset to keep your hands free without cramping your neck.

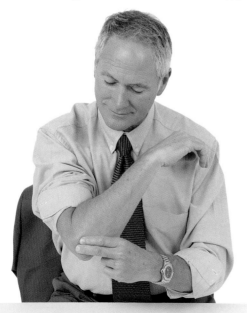

7 Bring your hand to your elbow. Use the flat of your thumb or fingers to make circular rotations around the joint, changing hand positions, as necessary.

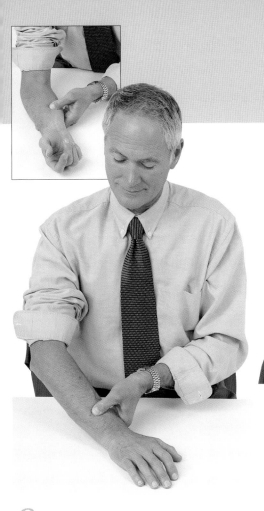

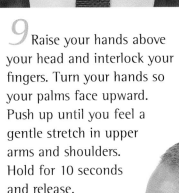

9 Raise your hands above your head and interlock your fingers. Turn your hands so your palms face upward. Push up until you feel a gentle stretch in upper arms and shoulders. Hold for 10 seconds and release.

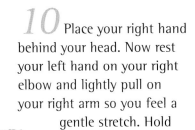

10 Place your right hand behind your head. Now rest your left hand on your right elbow and lightly pull on your right arm so you feel a gentle stretch. Hold for 5–10 seconds. Repeat on the other side.

8 Now use your thumb to make static pressures along your outer forearm. If it is more comfortable, use the pads of first or second fingers. Begin a little way up from the wrist (this area is too delicate for deep pressures). Press into the muscle with your thumb, hold for a count of 3, and release. Move along your forearm and repeat. Cover the whole of your outer forearm. Soothe the whole area, including the wrist, with gentle stroking.

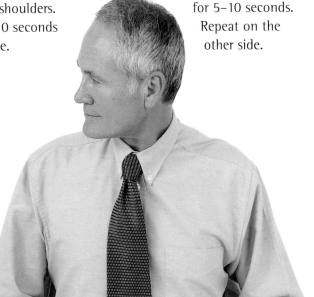

11 Bring your arms down by your sides with shoulders relaxed and hands resting comfortably in front of you. Slowly turn your head to look over your right shoulder. Do not force the stretch— only move as far as you comfortably can. Hold for a count of 5. Now turn your head to look over your left shoulder. Hold for a count of 5. Bring your head back to the center to look ahead. Repeat 3 times.

Memory lapses

Do you often find it difficult to remember names? Does it take longer to learn new facts? Do you find yourself repeating the same stories? Most people find that certain aspects of their memory start to decline after age 50. However, there is plenty you can do to boost brain power —whatever your age.

This simple 5-minute massage sequence can boost the flow of blood, oxygen, and nutrients to the brain, encouraging the cells concerned with memory to work to their full potential.

1 Using your finger pads, tap across your forehead and over your temples. Continue tapping all over your scalp.

2 Place both hands on the hairline above your forehead. Cup your hands and splay out your fingers. Press firmly with the tips of your fingers and thumbs. Hold for a count of 5 and release. Move your hands a little way back and repeat. Continue until you have covered your whole head with firm fingertip pressures.

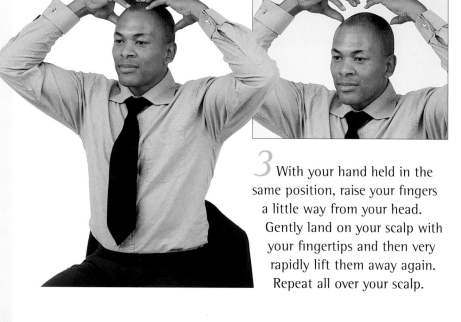

3 With your hand held in the same position, raise your fingers a little way from your head. Gently land on your scalp with your fingertips and then very rapidly lift them away again. Repeat all over your scalp.

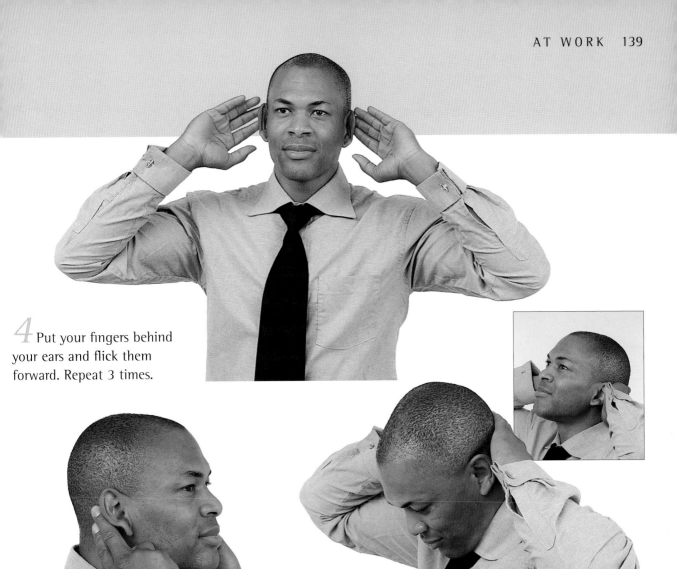

4 Put your fingers behind your ears and flick them forward. Repeat 3 times.

5 Now circle your ears with the pads of your first and second fingers. Move in a counterclockwise direction, gradually increasing the speed. Choose a pressure and speed that feel good for you. Complete about 15 circles.

6 Rest your hands behind your neck, fingers firmly interlocking and elbows raised. Lower your head, and allow the weight of your arms to draw your chin down toward your chest. Release the pressure of your hold and raise your head. Repeat, this time making a long, controlled exhalation as you slowly lower your head. Inhale as you return to the starting position. Repeat once more. Bring your hands down by your sides. Now test yourself: Can you remember that forgotten name?

TECHNIQUE CHECKLIST

◆ Tapping ◆ Pressures ◆ Stroking ◆ Stretching (see pages 38–55)

Stiff neck and shoulders

The adult head weighs 6½–11 pounds (3–5 kg). Just think how hard the neck and shoulders have to work to support it. The weight puts a huge strain on the neck and shoulder muscles, leading to tension, stiffness, and discomfort.

This sequence of self-massage moves takes only 5–10 minutes and helps mobilize the joints, relax the muscles, and boost circulation to the head, neck, and shoulders. It can be performed while sitting in an office chair. The sequence is even more effective if you take a short walk around the office before and after.

1 Sit in your office chair. Start to ease the tension in your shoulders with this simple exercise. Hold your arms out from your body, palms facing upward. Keeping your elbows straight, rotate your arms so the palms are downward. Feel the movement in your shoulder joints.

2 With your arms hanging loosely by your sides, bring your shoulders right up to your ears, and hold for a count of 5. Let them drop down as far as you can. Try releasing an exaggerated sigh as you lower your shoulders.

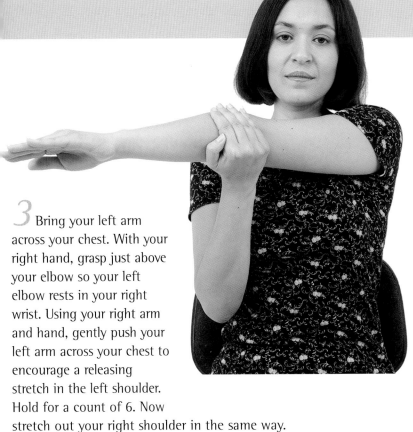

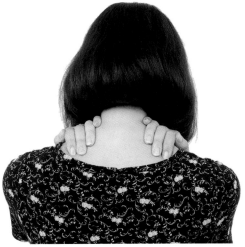

3 Bring your left arm across your chest. With your right hand, grasp just above your elbow so your left elbow rests in your right wrist. Using your right arm and hand, gently push your left arm across your chest to encourage a releasing stretch in the left shoulder. Hold for a count of 6. Now stretch out your right shoulder in the same way.

4 Place your hands on top of your shoulders. Knead the fleshy area here between your fingers and the heel of your hand. Continue for as long as you wish.

5 With your hands still on the tops of your shoulders, make firm pressures with 2 fingers along the muscles on the tops of your shoulders. Place the second fingers on top of the first fingers to reinforce the pressure. Press, hold for a count of 3, and then release. Move your fingers along until the whole area has been massaged. Repeat on the other side. →

TOP TIPS

◆ Check your sitting position when working at a computer to avoid neck and shoulder tension. Your chair and desk should be at the correct height so that your wrists are level with—or lower than—your elbows. Sit square to the computer screen so you do not have to twist to view it. Place your feet flat on the ground, legs uncrossed. Use a footrest if your feet do not reach the floor. Ensure that your back is straight and your lower back is well supported.

TECHNIQUE CHECKLIST

◆ Stretching ◆ Kneading ◆ Pressures ◆ Rubbing (see pages 38–55)

Stiff neck and shoulders...continued

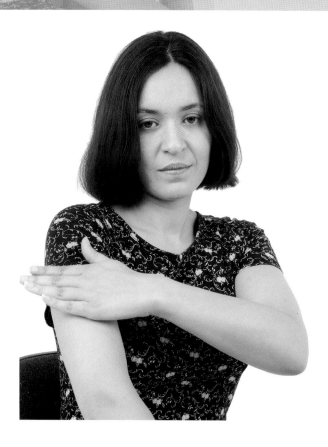

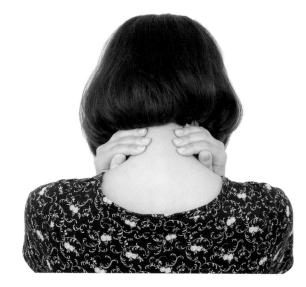

7 To relax the muscles in your neck, place your fingers on the soft tissue on either side of the vertebrae at the back of your neck. Use the fingertips of both hands to make small, gentle rotations up and down the back of your neck. Avoid applying too much pressure to this delicate area.

6 With the flat of your left hand, use a brisk rubbing action from the base of your neck, along the top of your right shoulder, and down your right arm. Keep the pressure fairly firm and avoid working over the same area for too long. When you reach your elbow, return to your shoulder and repeat. Change hands and work on your left shoulder.

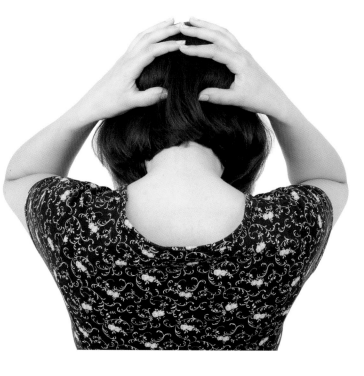

8 Lower your head a little and use your thumbs to apply pressure along the bony ridge of your skull. Repeat the movement, working outward to your ears. Repeat 3 times, slowly easing the muscular tension in this area.

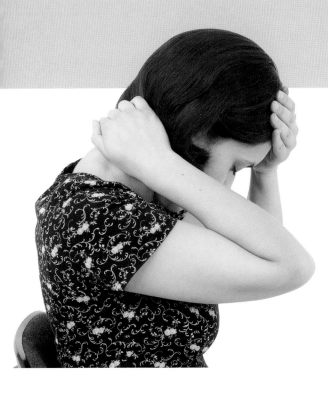

9 Place your right hand on the back of your neck, your palm molded to the shape of your neck. Hold your left hand on your head for support. Lower your head slightly and gently knead your neck, rolling the flesh between your fingers and the heel of your hand. Repeat, using the other hand.

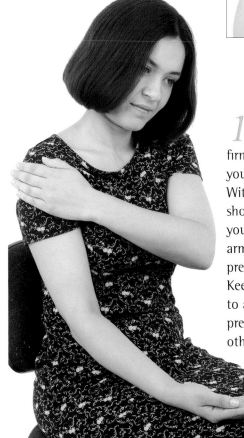

TOP TIPS

◆ If you are prone to neck tension, try wearing a scarf or turtleneck sweater. The warmth helps maintain a healthy blood circulation and keeps the muscles relaxed.

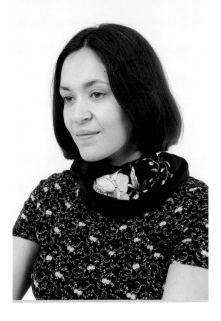

10 Finish the sequence with firm stroking movements from your neck down to your elbow. With your left hand on your right shoulder, stroke along the top of your shoulder, down your right arm to your elbow. Release the pressure and repeat 3 times. Keep the hand soft and relaxed to apply a firm but comfortable pressure. Repeat with the other arm.

Jaw ache

Most of us store tension in the jaw area without even realizing it. It is only when we start to suffer aches, pains, and stiffness in the jaw that we realize we may be habitually clenching our jaw muscles or grinding our teeth, often because of stress. These habits can become so ingrained that we even do them in our sleep.

This 5-minute self-massage sequence can help warm, relax, and soften the jaw muscles.

TOP TIPS

◆ Try dropping your lower jaw; then roll it from side to side to help relax tight muscles in the area.

1 Gently rub the fleshy area of your cheeks with the flats of two or more fingers. Use one hand at a time in a light back-and-forth upward rubbing action to warm and relax the muscles.

2 Now open and close your mouth. With your hands placed on your cheeks, feel for the muscles that make this movement. Once you have located the area, relax your mouth and press on it gently with the flats of two or more fingers. Now move the skin in large, slow circles. Maintain contact throughout the rotation without pressing too hard. Make 5 circles. Repeat on the other side.

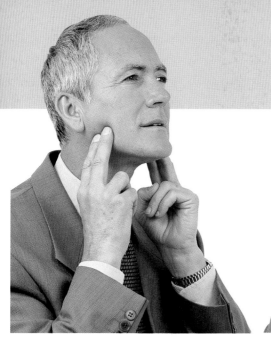

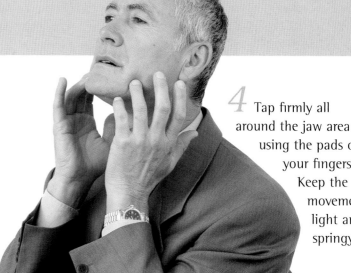

4 Tap firmly all around the jaw area using the pads of your fingers. Keep the movement light and springy.

3 Next make smaller rotations using the pads of two fingers all around your jaw area. Feel for any taut muscles and try to release the tension through massage. Keep the pressure firm but not uncomfortable.

TOP TIPS

◆ Periodically, check for jaw tension—maybe while sitting in a traffic jam or making a difficult telephone call. Make a conscious effort to relax your jaw. Is your mouth tightly closed? Open it so that your lips are just touching. Is your tongue on the roof of your mouth? Bring it to the center.

◆ Yawning is a great way of letting go of all the tension stored in your jaw. Better still, find a place where no one can hear you, then open your mouth widely and shout "Aaaah." This is a wonderful tension buster.

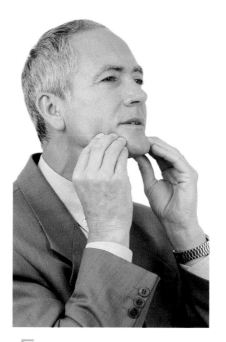

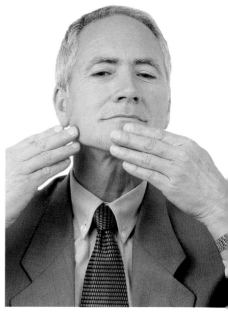

5 Gently squeeze the flesh along your lower jaw with the thumbs and first fingers of both hands. Start at your chin and work out toward your ears. Repeat 3 times.

6 Soothe the jaw area by gently stroking the pads of your fingers across your cheeks and under your chin. Keep your touch very soft. Stroke with both hands simultaneously or one after the other, whichever feels best.

TECHNIQUE CHECKLIST

◆ Rubbing ◆ Kneading ◆ Tapping ◆ Stroking (see pages 38–55)

Tired hands

Our hands work continuously, day in, day out. The many repetitive movements they perform can cause stiffness, pain, and fatigue. But massaging your hands regularly can help ease any buildup of tension, encourage joint mobility, and refresh tired, aching hands.

This simple sequence of moves requires no oils, takes only 5–10 minutes, and can be done easily at your desk, kitchen table, or using the arm of your chair.

1 Begin by warming your hands. Place your palms together. Move them against each other in a circular motion with the heel of one hand exerting the pressure. Continue for about 20 seconds or longer. Repeat, with the other hand leading the action. Keep the movement slow and rhythmical.

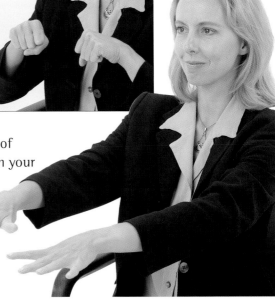

2 Make soft fists with both hands. Then quickly separate your fingers and thumbs and stretch them out as far as you can reach. Hold for a count of 5–10. Feel the tension in your fingers. Slowly release and return to soft fists. Repeat 3 times.

3 Put your left elbow on a desk or chair arm. Put the right thumb on your left arm, fingers beneath. Make small circular moves with the thumb from wrist to elbow. Slide back to the wrist. Repeat 6 times. Repeat on the right arm.

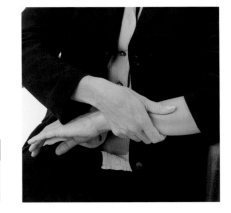

TECHNIQUE CHECKLIST

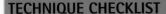 Rubbing 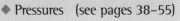 Kneading ◆ Stroking ◆ Pressures (see pages 38–55)

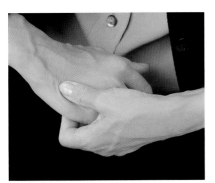

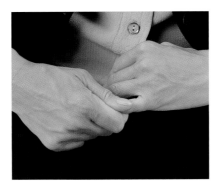

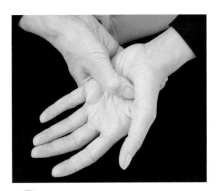

4 Support one hand, palm downward, in the fingers of the other hand. Now use the pad of your thumb to make small, circular kneading movements down the groove between the third and little fingers, working toward the wrist. Maintain skin contact, feeling for areas of tension. Repeat along the other grooves on top of the hand. Repeat on the other hand.

5 With your hand held palm downward, grasp the little finger between the thumb and forefinger of the other hand. Gently squeeze and massage along the finger with small circular movements. Move from the base of the finger to the tip. When your hand reaches the tip, give a gentle pull. Repeat this movement on all the fingers and thumb of one hand, and then on the other hand.

6 Turn your hand over to massage your palm. With your fingers supporting the back of your hand, use the pad of your thumb to make deep circular movements over the whole of your palm. Pay special attention to the muscular pad at the base of the thumb. Repeat on the other hand.

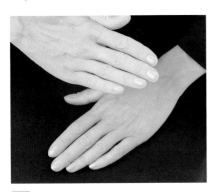

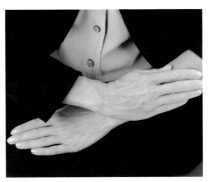

7 Now rest one hand on your knees, palm facing downward. Use the flat side of the fingers of the other hand to tap the back of the hand and fingers with light rapid movements. Turn your hand over and continue the springy movements across the palm and fingers. Repeat on the other hand.

8 Finish the sequence with long, firm stroking movements from the tips of the fingers to the elbow. When you reach the elbow, release the pressure and glide your hand back to the starting position. Keep your hand soft and relaxed as you do the movement. Continue for as long as you wish.

TOP TIPS

◆ Keep your hands soft and supple by using this massage sequence when putting moisturizer on your hands. Keep hand cream in several different places to remind you.

◆ Whenever your hands feel tired, stop what you are doing and shake them to ease any stiffness and to encourage blood flow to the fingers.

◆ While massaging your hands, take deep, calming breaths to relieve any mental and physical tension.

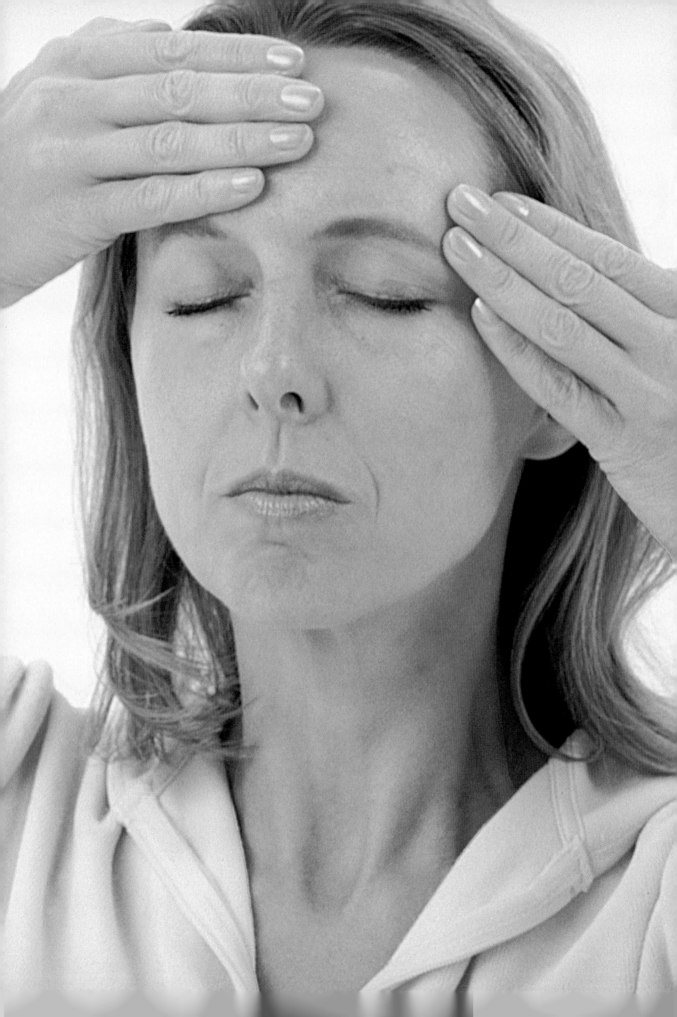

6 THE PROGRAMS

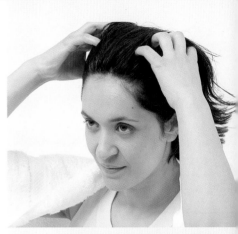

With regular daily or weekly stress-busting massage sessions, you'll find the benefits abound. As physical and emotional tension eases, you'll find your energy levels increasing and your sleep patterns improving. So set aside time to follow these simple self-massage programs designed to fit smoothly into your busy lifestyle. Try waking up to an energizing massage or going to bed with a soothing, sleepy massage. Once you start to reap the rewards, you'll soon find that self-massage becomes an integral part of your everyday routine.

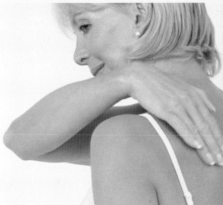

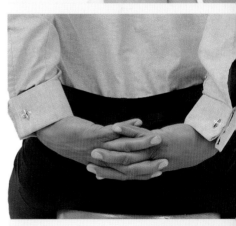

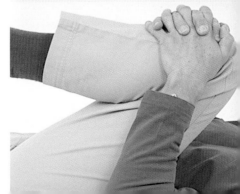

program 1 · Boost your circulation

Efficient circulation is essential for general health and vitality. When blood circulation is sluggish, energy levels start to fall, muscles may feel stiff and cold, and it is harder to stay focused. This 10-to-15-minute 12-step stretching and massage routine is an ideal morning wake-up call. Use a stable chair for support and give yourself plenty of space to allow you to make the most of the stretches.

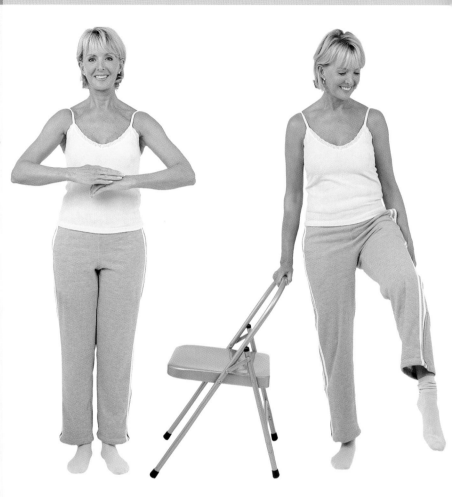

1 Begin by warming your hands. Rub them together—palm to palm, top of hand to palm, and fingers to fingers. Start to feel the heat as this simple, natural movement stimulates the blood circulation.

2 Hold on to a wall or chair for support (or place your hands on your hips) and raise your left foot a little way off the floor. Let your left leg feel soft and floppy; then gently shake it out. Turn your body and repeat with the right leg.

TECHNIQUE CHECKLIST

◆ Stretching ◆ Stroking ◆ Tapping ◆ Beating ◆ Rubbing (see pages 38–55)

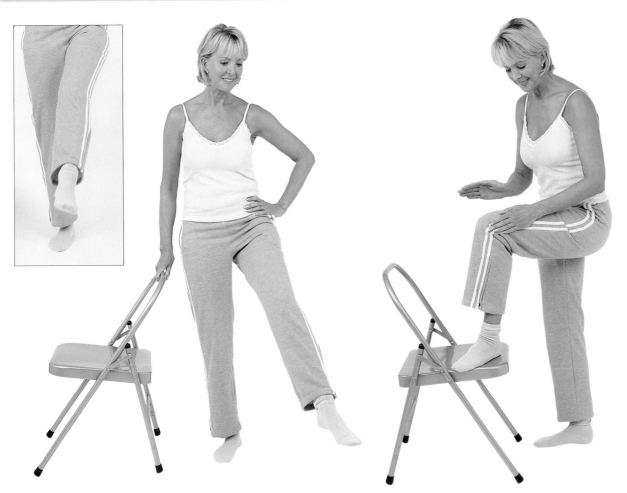

3 Still standing in the same position, raise your left foot a little way from the floor and trace a circle with your foot. Make the circle as large as feels comfortable for you. Do not force the action. Feel the movement coming from your hip. Make about 3 circles in one direction and 3 in the other direction. Repeat with your right leg.

4 Prop one leg on a stable chair. Gently tap your leg using the flats of both hands in an alternate rhythm, working from your calf up to your thigh. As one hand lands on the flesh, the other bounces back. Continue over your whole leg in an upward direction, moving around so you do not remain in the same spot for too long. Repeat with other leg.

5 Reach your hands as far down your left leg as feels comfortable. Now stroke firmly upward with the flats of your hands, one hand moving after the other in a series or wavelike strokes covering the entire leg. The strokes can be any length, as long as they move in an upward direction toward the heart.   →

program 1

Boost your circulation...continued

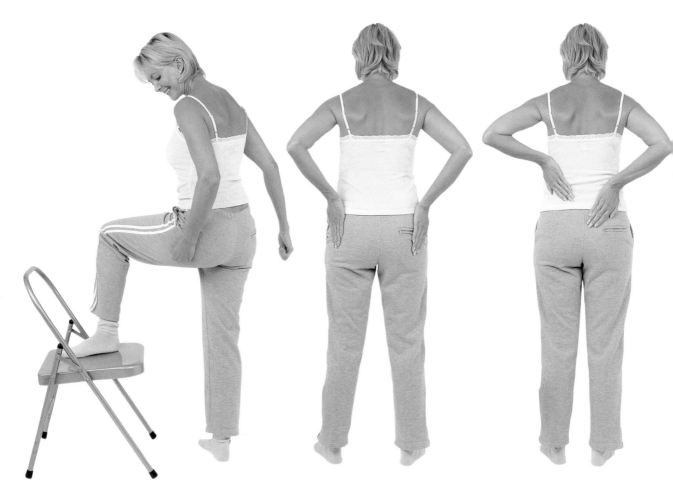

6 With hands held in a loose fist, place your left hand on your left buttock and right hand on your right buttock. Using the flats of your fingers and heels of your hands, gently beat the whole of this fleshy area. Your hands work simultaneously, building up a steady rhythm and increasing the pressure. Repeat Step 5 continuing the strokes over your buttocks.

7 Put both feet flat on the floor again. Lean forward slightly and place the flats of your hands on your lower back. Stroke your palms in big, circular movements over this area. Begin slowly and then gradually increase speed.

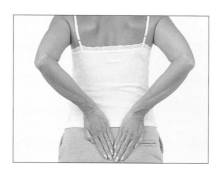

8 Keeping your hands behind your back, stand up straight. Now stroke firmly over your lower back with the flats of your hands working alternately. Continue the strokes as far up your back as you can. As one stroke finishes, the other begins. Do not overstretch on this move; keep within your own comfort zone.

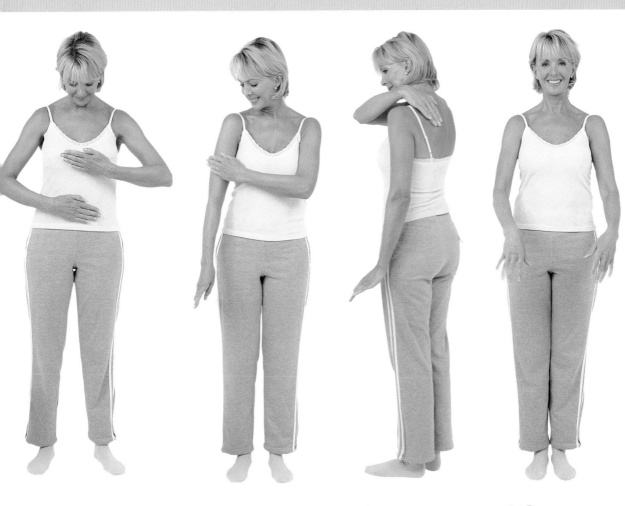

9 Continue the upward stroking action around your waist and over your abdomen. Change hands so you can work all the way around your body.

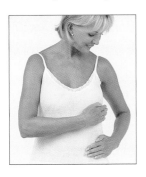

10 Using the flats of the fingers of your left hand, rub up your right arm from your wrist to your shoulder and across your chest. (The same stroking action as in Step 9.) Keep your fingers stiff and wrist flexible to produce a brisk back-and-forth action. Repeat on other side.

11 Now try taking your right hand over the left shoulder to rub your upper back, and vice versa, and then rub your scalp. Take care not to overstretch.

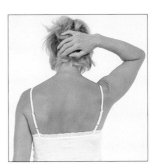

12 Complete the sequence by shaking your arms and then bringing them down to hang loosely by your sides. Can you feel a tingling sensation now that your circulation has been given a boost?

Start the morning with this daily 10-minute 11-step routine. Stretching and massaging your hands is such a wonderful way of encouraging joint mobility. You may find it more comfortable to support your elbows for some of the movements, so try doing the program in bed or at the breakfast table.

WARNING
If you have arthritis or another joint condition that affects your hands and arms, seek the advice of your doctor or physical therapist before trying these exercises.

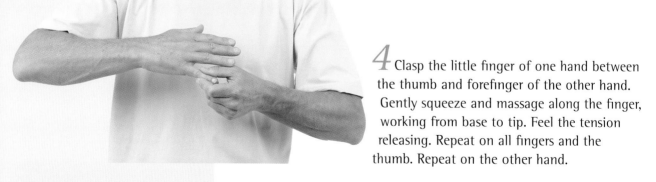

1 Place the palms of your hands together in "prayer" position. Press your hands firmly together. Hold for a count of 5. Gently push out your knuckle joints to form a diamond shape with your hands. Hold for a count of 5. Release and repeat 3 times.

4 Clasp the little finger of one hand between the thumb and forefinger of the other hand. Gently squeeze and massage along the finger, working from base to tip. Feel the tension releasing. Repeat on all fingers and the thumb. Repeat on the other hand.

TECHNIQUE CHECKLIST

◆ Stretching   ◆ Kneading   ◆ Stroking   ◆ Feathering   (see pages 38–55)

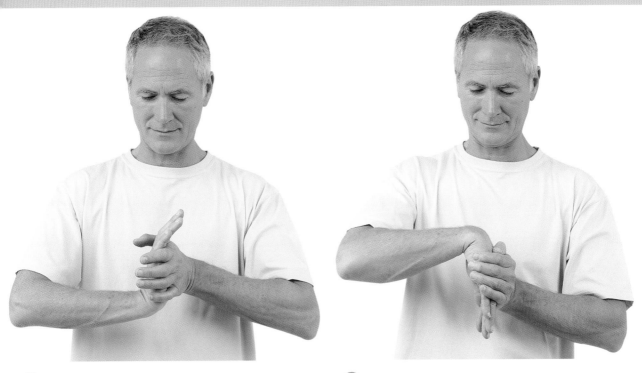

2 With hands at chest height, grasp your right palm in your left palm. Using your left hand to exert a slight pressure, bend your right hand back as far as is comfortable. Hold for a count of 3. Release.

3 Now push your hand downward with fingers stretching toward the floor. Hold for a count of 3. Release.

5 Begin in the same position as the previous step. Now gently pull to give the whole finger a good stretch. Hold for a count of 5. Release your hold and glide your hand along the finger, slowly floating off the tip. This feels great in the morning. Repeat on all fingers and thumb.   ➔

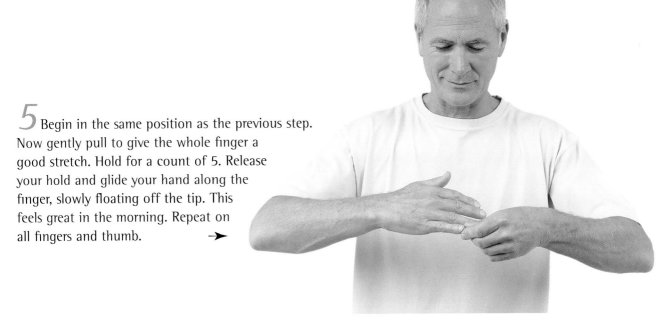

program2 Exercise your hands...continued

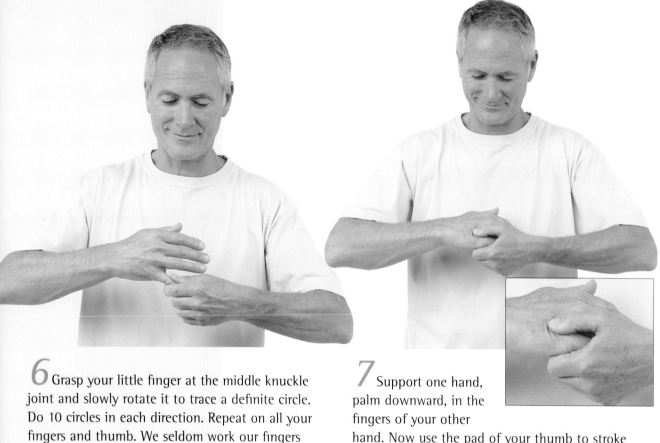

6 Grasp your little finger at the middle knuckle joint and slowly rotate it to trace a definite circle. Do 10 circles in each direction. Repeat on all your fingers and thumb. We seldom work our fingers independently, and this is a useful exercise to help prevent joint stiffness.

7 Support one hand, palm downward, in the fingers of your other hand. Now use the pad of your thumb to stroke firmly and evenly down the groove between each tendon on the hand, working from the knuckles to the wrist. Repeat. Now repeat with the other hand.

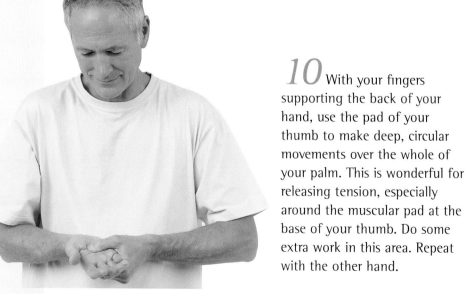

10 With your fingers supporting the back of your hand, use the pad of your thumb to make deep, circular movements over the whole of your palm. This is wonderful for releasing tension, especially around the muscular pad at the base of your thumb. Do some extra work in this area. Repeat with the other hand.

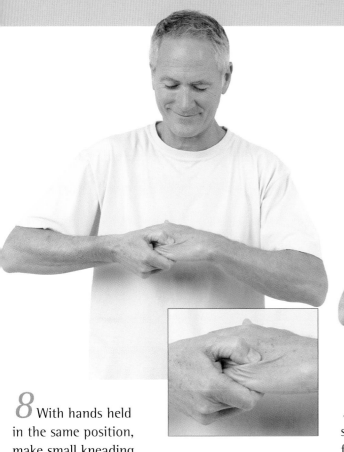

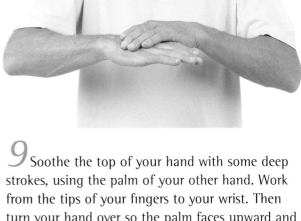

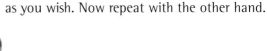

8 With hands held in the same position, make small kneading rotations with your thumb along the grooves on the top of your hand. Use a comfortably firm pressure, feeling for any areas of tension. Now repeat with the other hand.

9 Soothe the top of your hand with some deep strokes, using the palm of your other hand. Work from the tips of your fingers to your wrist. Then turn your hand over so the palm faces upward and repeat the stroking action. Continue for as long as you wish. Now repeat with the other hand.

11 Finish with gentle featherlike strokes on the wrist. Using the thumb, stroke with a gentle, circular motion. Cover the whole of the outer wrist, keeping the pressure light on this delicate area. Skin should not move under your light touch. Turn the hand over and repeat the circular stroking on your inner wrist. Repeat with the other hand.

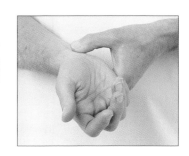

program 3

Warm up for work

How does your workday usually begin? Take a tip from Asia, where office workers are encouraged to warm up before they start work. This simple 10-step routine takes less than 10 minutes and can be performed in your office chair.

Try to get into work a few minutes early so you can practice the sequence when you have the office to yourself.

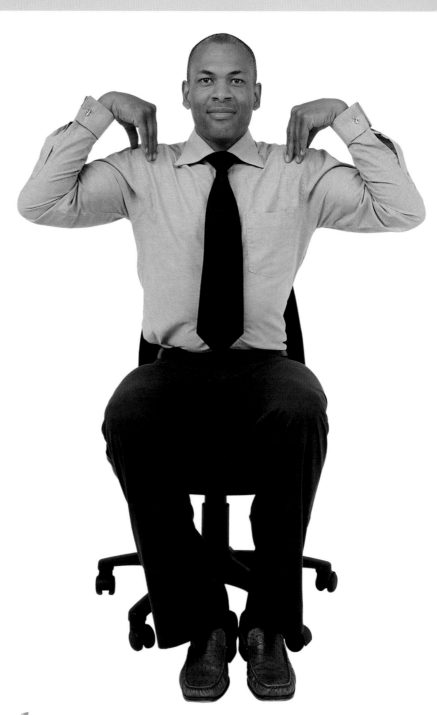

1 Begin by sitting comfortably, legs uncrossed and hands hanging loosely by your sides. Now place your hands on your shoulders. Circle your elbows backward in a slow, controlled movement. Do 5 circles. Now repeat the circles in a forward direction. Feel the release of tension in your shoulders and upper back.

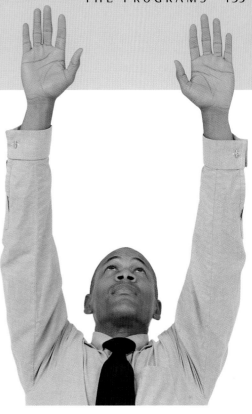

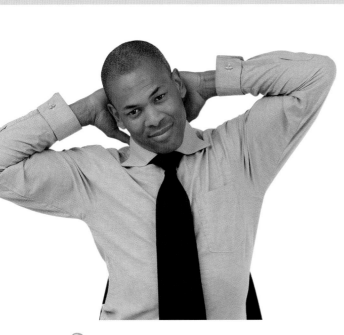

2 Gently cradle the back of your head with both hands, fingers interlocking and elbows to the sides. Tilt your neck to one side so that your right ear moves toward your right shoulder. Hold for a count of 5. Bring your head upright and then slowly allow your head to lean to the other side. Hold for a count of 5. Repeat 3 times.

3 Hold both arms straight up above your head. Stretch up with your hands as far as you can reach. Hold for a count of 5 and release.

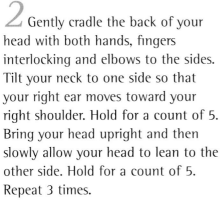

4 With your hands still above your head, trace 10 small circles with your arms, first in one direction and then in the other direction. Bring your hands back down to your sides. →

program3   Warm up for work...continued

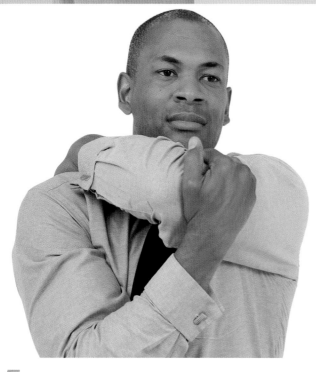

5 Raise your left arm and bend the elbow so that your hand reaches down your neck to your upper back. Hold the elbow with the right hand and pull gently for a count of 5. Feel a releasing stretch in the upper arm. Relax and repeat on the other arm. Repeat 3 times.

6 Clasp your hands behind you, with fingers interlocked. Bend your elbows and press your upper arms inward, so you feel a squeeze between your shoulder blades. Release and repeat 3 times.

9 This exercise promotes flexibility in your ankles. Rest your right ankle over your left knee. Hold your foot with one hand and support your ankle with the other. Gently rotate the ankle in a clockwise direction 10 times. Repeat in the other direction.

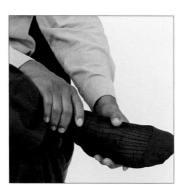

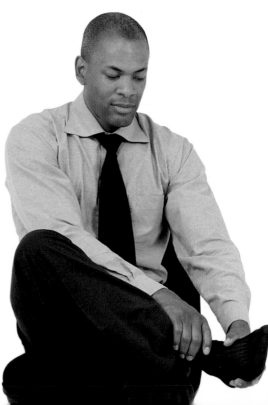

TECHNIQUE CHECKLIST

◆ Stretching   ◆ Rubbing   ◆ Kneading   ◆ Stroking

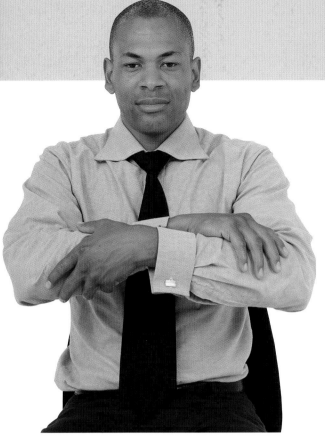

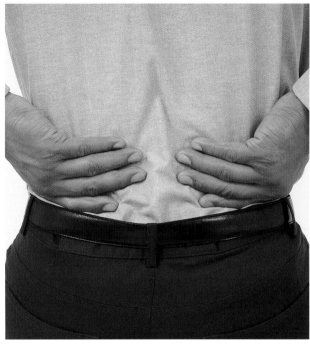

7 Clasp the opposite wrist with each hand. Bend your elbows and bring your hands to chest height. Push your hands toward your wrists in a fairly brisk back-and-forth rubbing action. Release when you reach the elbows. Repeat with arms at waist level and also at eye level.

8 Bring your hands to your lower back, and gently stroke and knead around the whole of this area with your fingers and palms. Continue around to your abdomen if you wish.

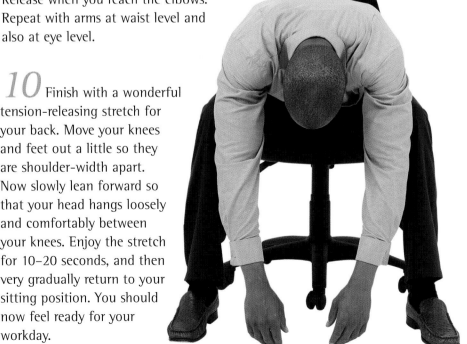

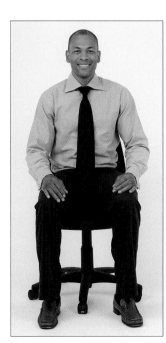

10 Finish with a wonderful tension-releasing stretch for your back. Move your knees and feet out a little so they are shoulder-width apart. Now slowly lean forward so that your head hangs loosely and comfortably between your knees. Enjoy the stretch for 10–20 seconds, and then very gradually return to your sitting position. You should now feel ready for your workday.

A soothing scalp-and-face massage can be very relaxing at the end of each day. This 11-step routine takes 10–15 minutes and is in two parts. The first part works on the scalp. The second part works on the face and neck—so you can apply night cream at the same time. Before you start, remove your makeup.

1 Begin by clearing your mind and calming your breathing. Sit upright in a chair with your hands in your lap. Close your eyes and concentrate on relaxing your shoulders and releasing any tense areas.

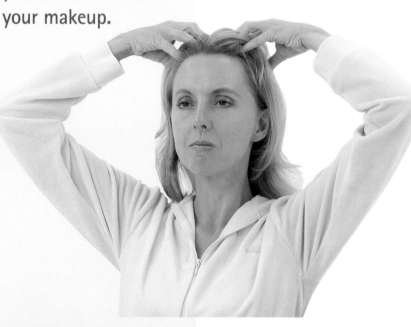

4 Continue to relax the muscles in your scalp. Place your hands on either side of your scalp with fingers in a wide, clawlike pose. Use the pads of the fingers and thumbs to make small circular movements all over the front, sides, and back of your head. Feel your scalp moving beneath your fingers.

TECHNIQUE CHECKLIST

◆ Holding   ◆ Kneading   ◆ Stroking   (see pages 38–55)

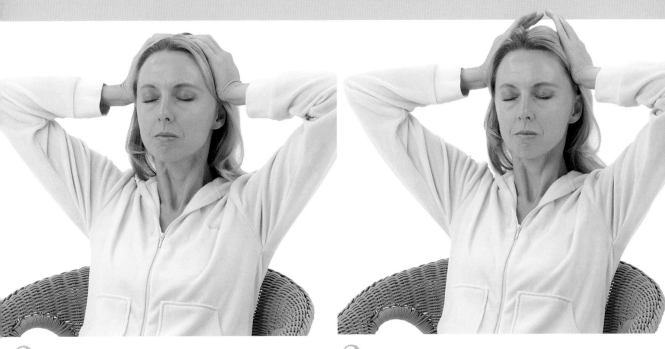

2 Cradle your head securely between your hands so the heels of your hands rest on your temples and your fingers meet at the top of your head. Exert as much pressure with your hands as feels comfortable. Hold for 1 minute. Repeat with the heels of your hands above your ears and then behind your ears.

3 With your hands on your head, fingers pointing upward, interlock your fingers and slowly press the palms of your hands inward and upward against your scalp so that the skin starts to move beneath your fingers. Move to another position and repeat. Do this move as often as you wish to release the tension trapped in your scalp.

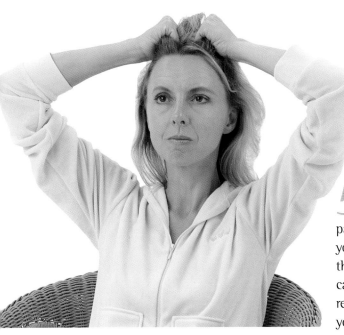

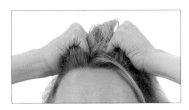

5 Push your fingers through your hair so the palms of your hands are resting on your scalp. Curl your fingers into fists, keeping your knuckles close to the scalp and getting hold of as much hair as you can. Gently tug on your hair. Imagine you are releasing the stresses of the day. Continue all over your head.

➜

program 4 Relax your face and scalp...cont.

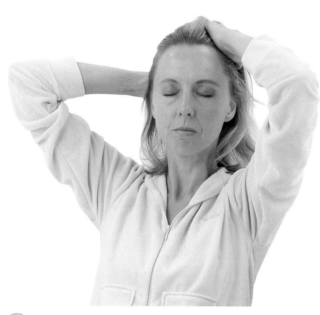

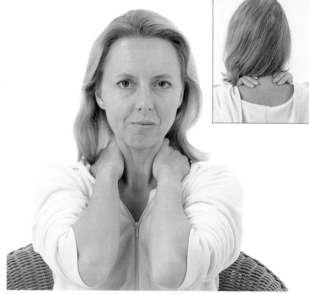

6 Smooth your hair back into place with long, flowing strokes from the hairline, back over the head to the neck. Use alternate hands so that as one hand finishes, the other starts in a continuous wavelike movement. Keep your hands and fingers soft and molded to the contours of your scalp.

7 Put the heels of your hands on your shoulders at the base of the neck, on either side of the spine. Massage in a kneading motion outward, across each shoulder.

Now clean your hands and apply your night cream with massage strokes all over your face and neck.

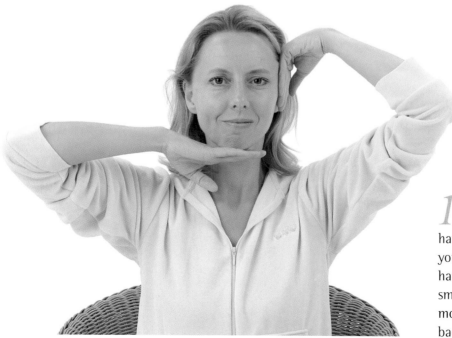

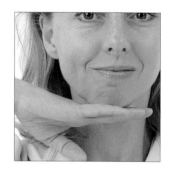

10 Use the backs of your hands to stroke up your neck to your jaw and cheeks. Glide one hand up after the other in a smooth, upward, flowing movement, working across and back to your ear.

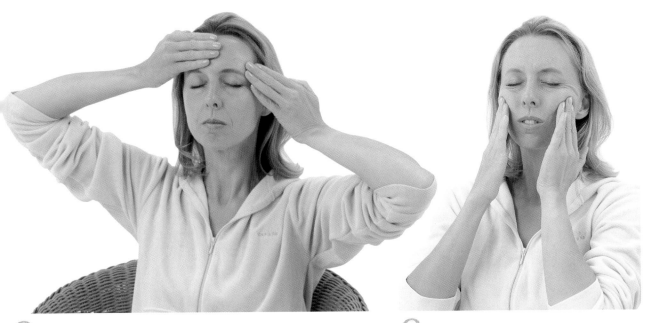

8 Start your face routine by soothing your brow. Place your fingers on your forehead. Use alternate hands to stroke from the center toward the temples in a flowing motion. Keep the movement very slow with a light, even pressure.

9 Move to the eye area. Use the pads of one or two fingers to stroke from the center of your brow along your eyebrows and around the top of your cheeks to form large, comforting circles around your eyes.

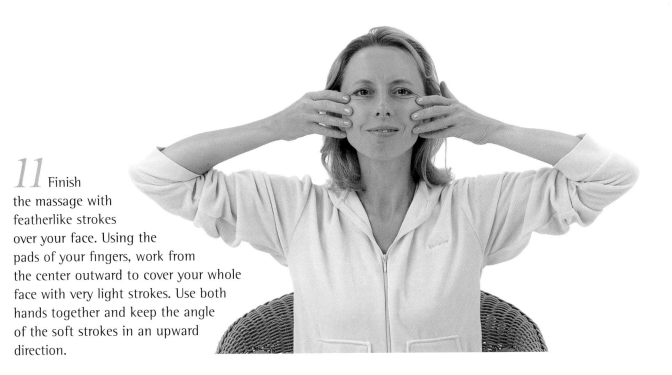

11 Finish the massage with featherlike strokes over your face. Using the pads of your fingers, work from the center outward to cover your whole face with very light strokes. Use both hands together and keep the angle of the soft strokes in an upward direction.

program5 Mind your back

It has been estimated that 4 out of 5 people will suffer back pain at some time in their lives. This simple 11-step daily stretching program helps keep your back strong and supple. Choose a comfortable surface, such as a carpet or an exercise mat. Support your neck with a small pillow or rolled-up towel, and keep your movements slow and controlled.

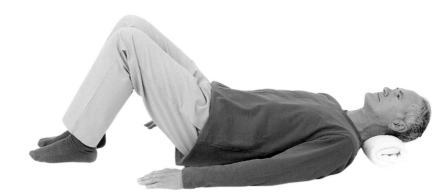

1 Begin by lying on the floor and placing a support under your neck. Bend your knees and place your hands by your sides. Tighten your tummy muscles so that you feel your back flatten against the floor. Hold for a count of 5. Repeat 3 times.

WARNING
Perform the stretches very gently. If you feel any pain, immediately stop this exercise.

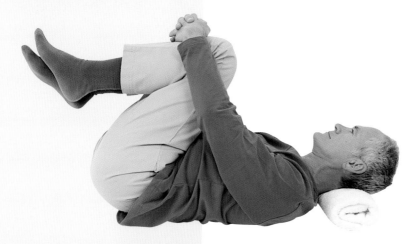

4 Staying in the same position, gently rock your back from side to side in a rhythmical, flowing motion. Continue for as long as feels good to help ease the tension that often builds up in the lower back muscles.

TECHNIQUE CHECKLIST

◆ Stretching   (see pages 38–55)

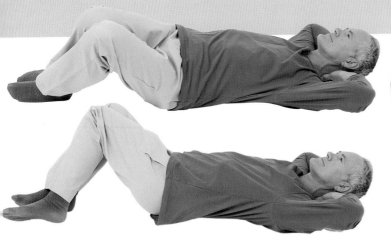

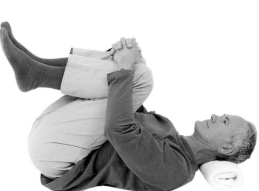

2 Gently clasp your hands behind your head. Bend your knees with your feet flat on the floor. Roll your knees to one side as far as they will comfortably go—do not force the stretch. Keep your knees together. Keep the movement slow and deliberate. Stay in the stretch for a count of 10. Repeat on each side 3 times for a count of 5.

3 Bring both knees to your chest and clasp them with your hands. Gently pull your knees toward your chest and enjoy the releasing stretch in your back. Hold for a count of 5. Release the pull, but continue holding your knees. Repeat.

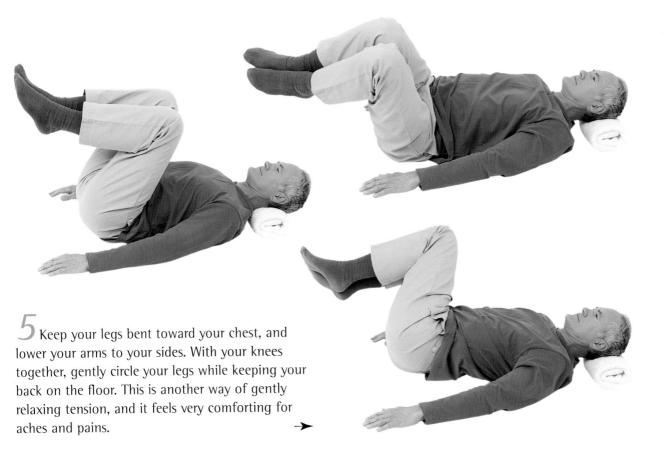

5 Keep your legs bent toward your chest, and lower your arms to your sides. With your knees together, gently circle your legs while keeping your back on the floor. This is another way of gently relaxing tension, and it feels very comforting for aches and pains.

→

program5 Mind your back...continued

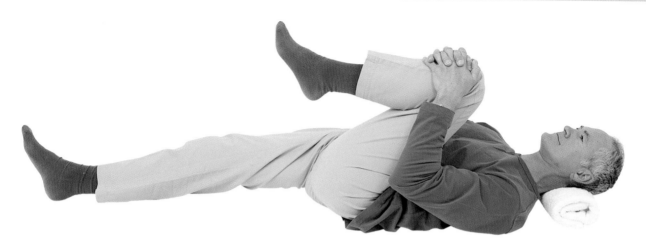

6 Lower your legs to the floor. Bend one leg and clasp the knee with your hands. Pull your bent leg very gently toward your chest as far as feels comfortable. Hold for a count of 5. Repeat with each leg 3 times.

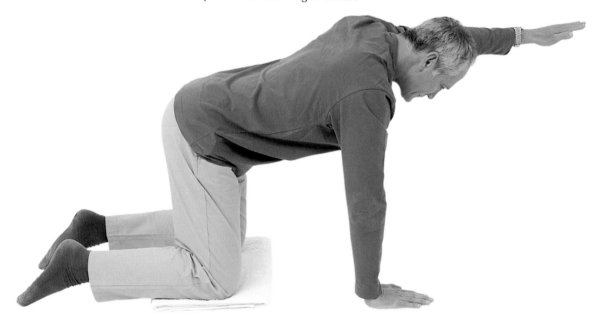

9 In the same starting position as Steps 7 and 8, tighten your tummy and raise one arm in front of you. Hold for a count of 10. Keep your body in line—be careful not to twist or turn. Repeat with the other arm. Repeat 5 times on each side.

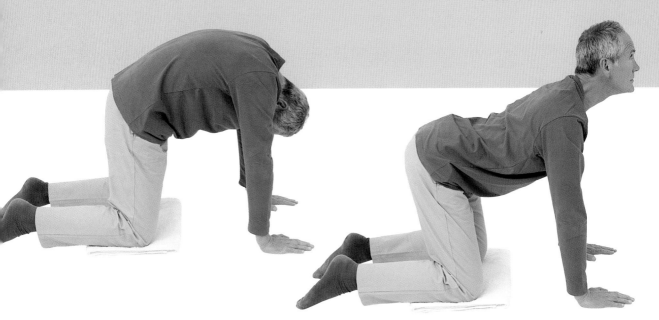

7 Get onto your hands and knees, with hands shoulder-width apart, arms and thighs vertical, and back parallel to the floor. Exhale, and round your back away from the floor. Look down at the floor. Hold for a count of 5.

8 Continue the stretch by inhaling and gently lowering your tummy toward the floor. Hollow your back and look up to the ceiling. Enjoy the stretch. Repeat this step and the previous step 5 times.

WARNING
If you are pregnant, avoid doing Step 8.

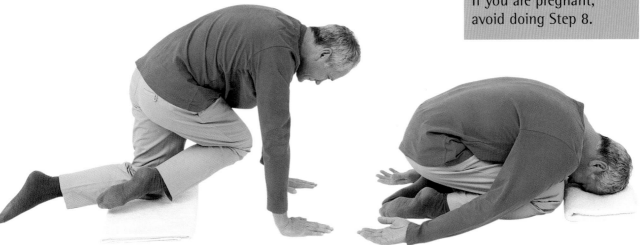

10 Draw your right knee toward your left elbow. Stretch only as far as you can without causing any discomfort. Hold for a count of 3 and release. Repeat with your right knee stretching toward your left elbow. Repeat 5 times.

11 Finish with a glorious stretch, known as the "child's pose" in yoga. Curl forward over your thighs to rest your forehead on the floor with your chin tucked in. Bring your hands alongside your feet, palms facing upward. Stay in this relaxing position for as long as you feel comfortable. If you feel any tightness, place a small pad or pillow between your feet and buttocks or under your forehead.

Give yourself a weekly head massage with natural oils. There is no need to wash your hair first. But if you do wash your hair, towel-dry and, in either case, comb through with a wide-toothed comb before massaging. For this 10-step massage you will need to use massage oil—sweet almond or jojoba are ideal (see Step 1).

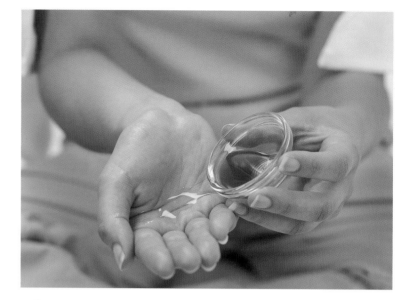

1 Wear old clothes and wrap a towel around your shoulders, as oil can splash and stain. Pour some oil into your palms and rub your hands together so they are warm and well covered in oil. The amount of oil will depend on the length and texture of your hair and your personal preference. Some people love to have their hair saturated in oil; others prefer just a little. You can keep topping up the oil as necessary.

4 Rub firmly and briskly all over your scalp. Using the pads of the fingers on one or both hands, start at the back of your ears and cover your whole head. Keep the fingers moving continuously in short side-to-side movements.

TECHNIQUE CHECKLIST

◆ Stroking   ◆ Kneading   ◆ Rubbing   ◆ Raking   (see pages 38–55)

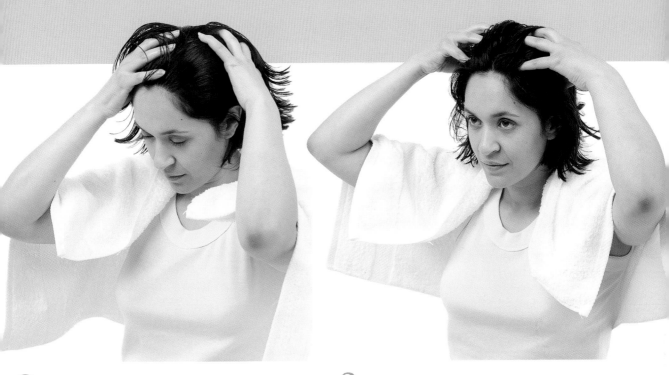

2 Starting from the front of your head and working toward the back, stroke the oil evenly all over your scalp and hair. Then stroke from the sides of your head to the crown, ensuring that your scalp and hair are completely covered in oil.

3 Place your hands in a clawlike position on your head, fingers well spread out, and make finger rotations with the pads of your fingers and thumbs all over your scalp. Experiment with both a lighter and firmer pressure to discover what feels best for you. Feel the scalp moving and relaxing beneath the kneading action of your fingers. Your hands should move continuously, and be moving across your entire scalp. Include the back of your head and behind your ears.

5 Place your hands in a loosely clenched fist and continue this rapid side-to-side rubbing movement, using the backs of your curled fingers to massage all over the scalp. This movement feels really good along the bony edge at the base of your skull. ➤

program6

Condition your hair...continued

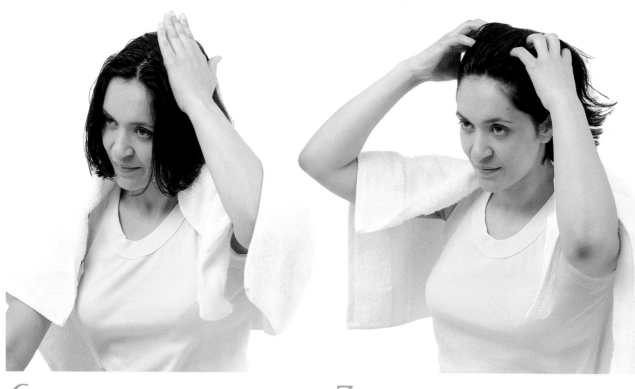

6 Continue this circulation-boosting sequence with a friction rub using the flat of one hand. Keeping the hand held fairly rigid, rub briskly until you have covered the whole scalp. Repeat using the other hand.

7 Now rake over your scalp. Curl your fingers and use your fingertips to "comb" your hair back in place. Work from the front of your head to the back. Enjoy the tingling sensation this move creates. Try raking with both hands together or one following the other in a flowing action. Continue for as long as you wish.

9 Complete the routine with smoothing strokes from the front of your head to the back. This helps soothe the area after the previous stimulating movements. Use these strokes to settle your hair back in place.

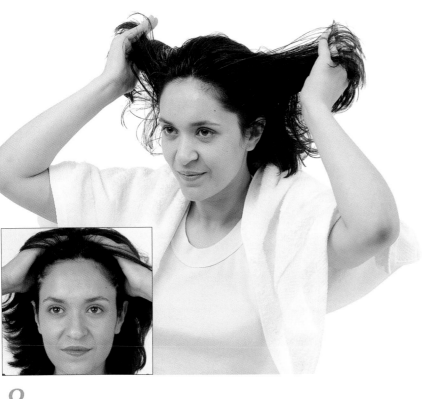

8 The next move involves gently pulling at the roots of your hair to help stimulate blood circulation to the scalp and encourage healthy hair growth. First draw your hands through your hair with your fingers spread out. Rest your hands in this position on the scalp. Now bring your fingers together so you grasp a handful of hair. Give a gentle pull. Release the hold and slide your fingers through your hair, drawing lightly away when you reach the tips. Continue over your whole head.

10 To finish, wrap a warm towel around your head and rest for at least 30 minutes. This allows time for the oil to penetrate and nourish your hair and scalp.

The first part of this 11-step program is wonderful for releasing the tension that can build up in the muscles of the head and neck as a result of stress. The second part helps you develop an awareness and control of your breathing pattern. When you breathe effectively, the movement comes from the diaphragm, not the chest. Allow 10–15 minutes for the whole program. Dress in loose clothing, remove your shoes, and sit upright.

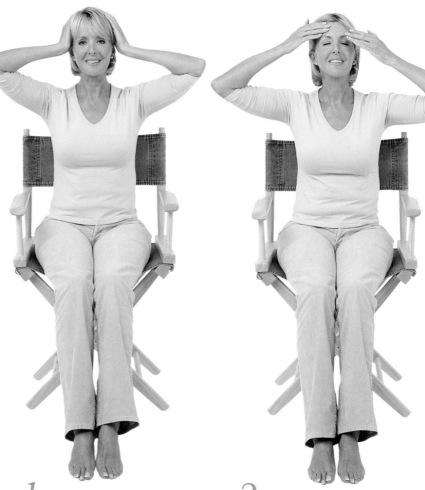

1 Bring your hands to your head. Cradle your head in the palms of your hands. Hold for at least 1 minute. Feel the comforting warmth of your hands encouraging a sense of stillness in mind and body.

2 Gently stroke your forehead with the tips of your fingers to help you relax. One hand moves after the other in a slow, rhythmic way. As your fingers stroke your skin softly, notice how your breathing slows.

TECHNIQUE CHECKLIST

◆ Stretching ◆ Stroking ◆ Kneading ◆ Holding (see pages 38–55)

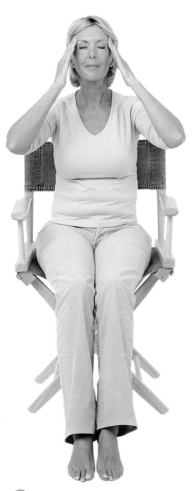

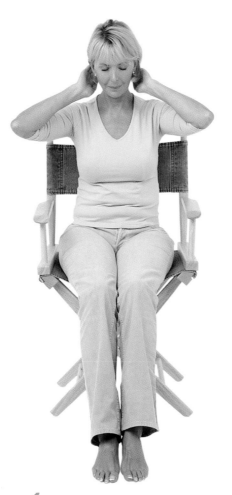

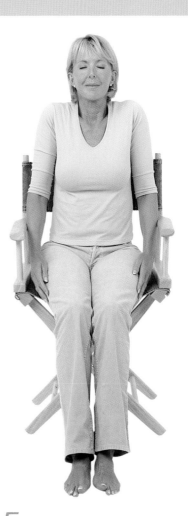

3 Place your hands on your temples. Using the pads of your first and second fingers, make slow, wide circular movements over the area. Feel the skin move beneath your touch as you gently ease out the tension. Make 10 circles in each direction. For best results, keep the movements slow.

4 Tilt your head forward a little. Bring both hands to the back of your neck and make small circular movements over the muscles here. Start at the base and work upward. Continue along the muscles that lie below the bone at the back of your scalp. Repeat using the other hand.

5 Now relax your shoulders. Raise both shoulders toward your ears. Hold for a count of 3. Release. ➔

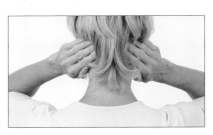

program 7 — Conquer your stress...continued

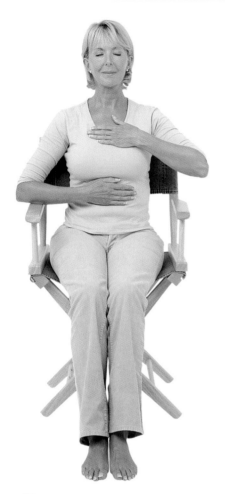

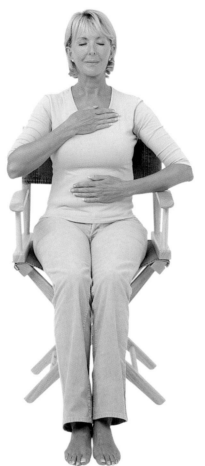

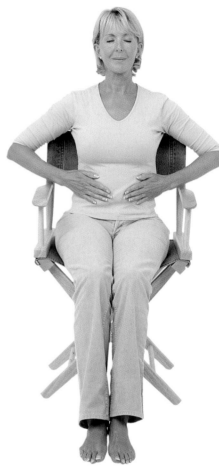

6 With your upper body relaxed, it is time to turn your attention to your breathing. Place one hand on your chest and the other on your abdomen, just below your breastbone. Hold your hands in this position. Breathe normally and notice which hand moves when you breathe. Ideally, your chest remains still and the hand on your abdomen rises and falls in a rhythmic way.

7 Alternate hands. Try taking a deeper breath so you can feel the movement coming from the diaphragm, not the chest, allowing the air to flow deep down into your lungs.

8 Place both hands just below your breastbone, fingers pointing inward but not touching. Take a slow, deep breath in through your nose to a count of 4, drawing the breath right down to your abdomen. As you inhale, be aware of your abdomen expanding as your diaphragm moves downward. Exhale slowly and gently through your nose for a count of 4. Concentrate on emptying your lungs. Pause for a few seconds. Repeat Steps 6 and 7, focusing on each breath as it enters and leaves your body.

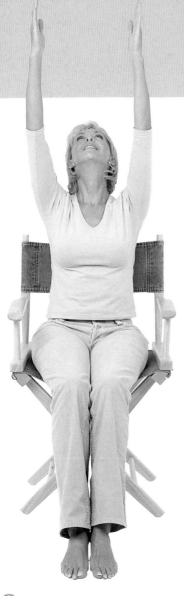

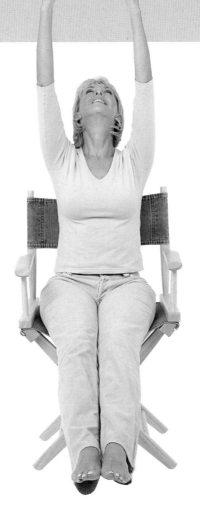

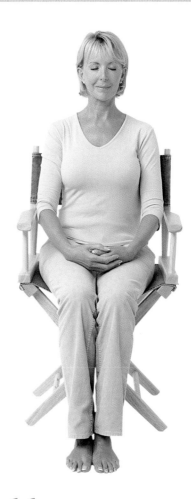

9 Remain sitting in a comfortable position. Breathe normally. Notice how relaxed you feel. When you are ready to come out of the relaxation, open your eyes and enjoy a good stretch. Raise both arms over your head and stretch up as far as you comfortably can. Yawn if you feel like it. Feel the stretch in your arms.

10 With your arms still extended, now stretch your legs, with toes pointing down and away from you. Hold for a count of 5. Release. Repeat.

11 Wait for 1–2 minutes before standing up. Do not hurry. Enjoy the feeling of peace and relaxation.

WARNING

If you feel faint or dizzy at any time during this breathing exercise, stop and return to your normal breathing pattern.

Regular full-body self-massage helps improve circulation, keeps skin in good condition, and soothes mental and physical tension. Depending on your mood and time restraints, this 12-step massage can take between 15 and 45 minutes. The best position to adopt is sitting on a towel or mat on the floor, with cushions or a wall to support your back. Sit with your legs crossed or stretched out in front.

1 Begin with your head. Using the flats of your fingers, gently tap all over your scalp and around your neck. Include your face if you wish. Keep your fingers moving so you do not stay on the same spot for too long.

4 Knead up your right arm, working from your wrist to the base of your neck. Using your left hand, pick up the flesh and gently squeeze it. Knead upward from your lower arm to your upper arm, covering the front and back of the arm. Repeat 3 times. Now repeat on the other arm.

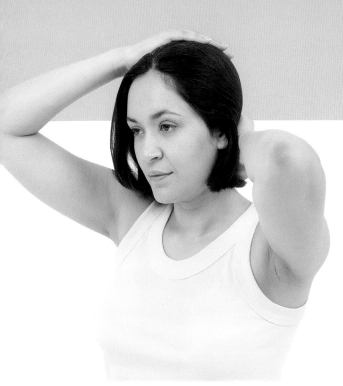

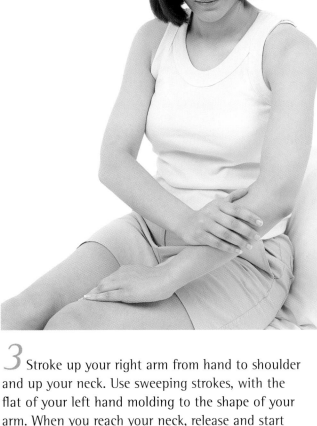

2 Now use alternate hands to stroke from the top of your head, down to your neck, and across the top of your shoulders. As one hand finishes the stroke, the next one begins. Keep your movements slow and rhythmical with long, flowing strokes.

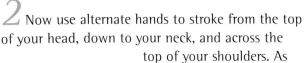

3 Stroke up your right arm from hand to shoulder and up your neck. Use sweeping strokes, with the flat of your left hand molding to the shape of your arm. When you reach your neck, release and start the stroking action again. Repeat 6 times, gradually applying a firmer pressure with each stroke. Repeat on the other arm.

5 Continue kneading over the tight band of muscle that runs across the tops of the shoulders. Continue for as long as feels comfortable. Finish this step with gentle strokes. The next stage is to work on the lower body.   →

TECHNIQUE CHECKLIST

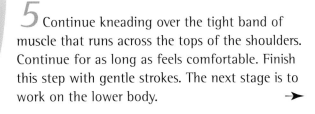

◆ Tapping   ◆ Stroking   ◆ Beating   ◆ Kneading   ◆ Pressures   (see pages 38–55)

program8 Tone from head to toe...continue

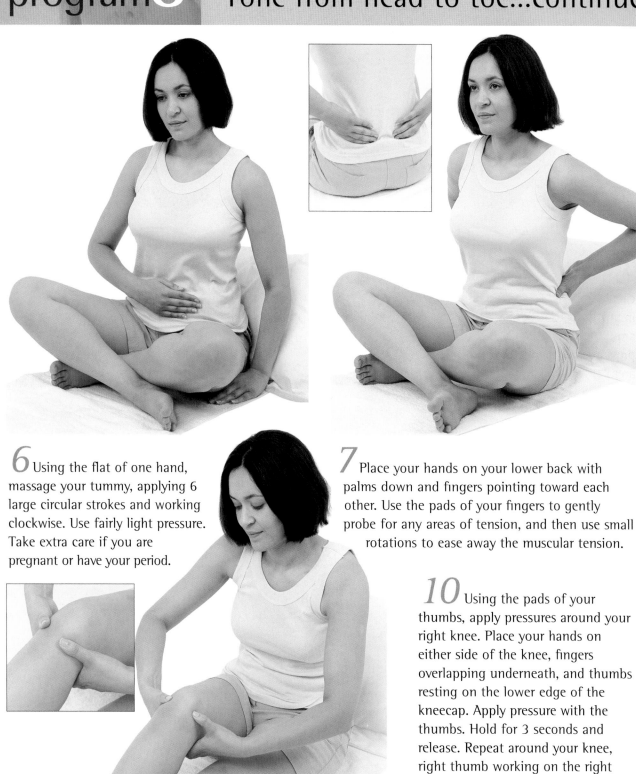

6 Using the flat of one hand, massage your tummy, applying 6 large circular strokes and working clockwise. Use fairly light pressure. Take extra care if you are pregnant or have your period.

7 Place your hands on your lower back with palms down and fingers pointing toward each other. Use the pads of your fingers to gently probe for any areas of tension, and then use small rotations to ease away the muscular tension.

10 Using the pads of your thumbs, apply pressures around your right knee. Place your hands on either side of the knee, fingers overlapping underneath, and thumbs resting on the lower edge of the kneecap. Apply pressure with the thumbs. Hold for 3 seconds and release. Repeat around your knee, right thumb working on the right side of the knee, left thumb on the left side, until meeting at the top. Repeat on the left knee.

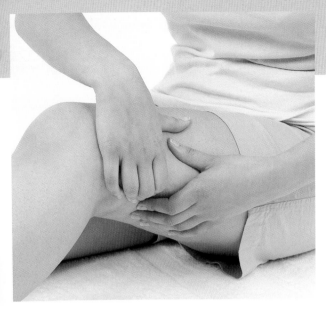

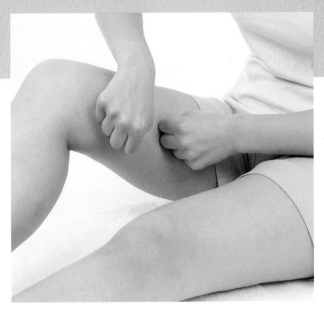

8 Now give your thighs a good workout to boost circulation and aid lymph drainage. Using both hands in an alternate kneading action, squeeze and pinch around your right thigh. Apply a firm but comfortable pressure, ensuring that you do not work over the same area for too long. Repeat on your left thigh.

9 Follow the kneading movement with beating. Hold your hands in loosely clenched fists and beat the flesh on your right thigh. This helps tone and firm the muscles. As one hand lands on the thigh, the other springs back. Start slowly, and gradually build up to a faster action. Repeat on your left thigh.

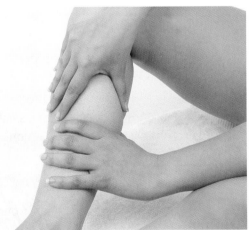

12 Finish by stroking the legs from toes to buttocks. Using the flat of your hand, make long, sweeping strokes upward. Include the front and back of the thigh. Stroke with both hands together or one after the other. Start firmly, gradually decreasing the pressure to featherlike strokes.

11 Bend your knee to massage your calf muscles, which often become tight and congested. Work from the ankle up to the knee, kneading the flesh between fingers and thumbs. Use one or both hands, whichever feels most comfortable.

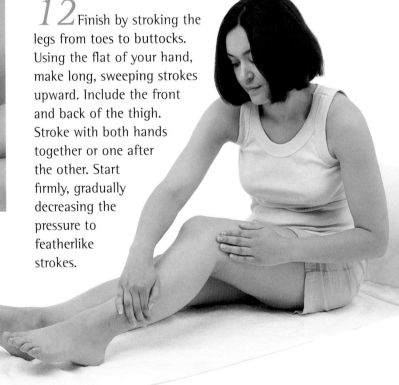

The soles of the feet are very sensitive; this explains why a weekly foot massage is such a good way to relax mind and body. Try mixing 1 teaspoon (5ml) of carrier oil with one drop of lavender essential oil. You need to be able to reach your foot comfortably, so sit on the floor, a chair, or a bed. Start with your right foot, then repeat on your left foot.

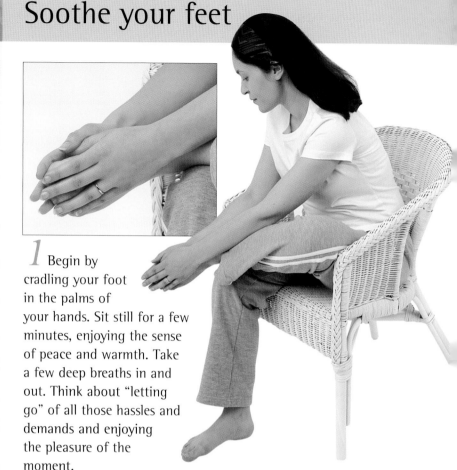

1 Begin by cradling your foot in the palms of your hands. Sit still for a few minutes, enjoying the sense of peace and warmth. Take a few deep breaths in and out. Think about "letting go" of all those hassles and demands and enjoying the pleasure of the moment.

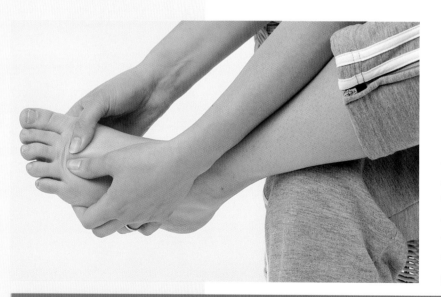

4 Place your fingers underneath your foot with your thumbs on top. Now gently knead around the top of your foot, making small circular movements with the pads of your thumbs. This feels particularly good at the base of your toes.

TECHNIQUE CHECKLIST

◆ Stroking   ◆ Tapping   ◆ Kneading   ◆ Stretching   ◆ Feathering   (see pages 38–55)

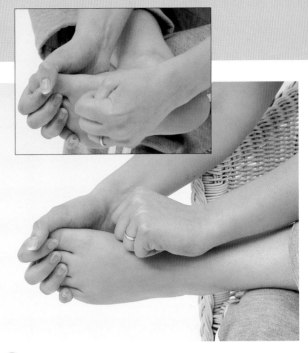

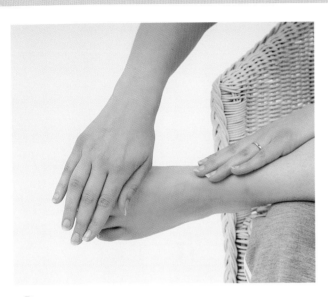

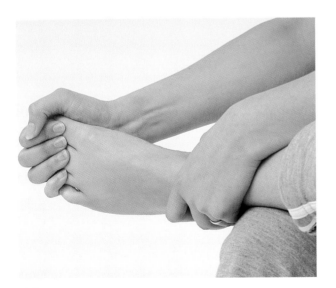

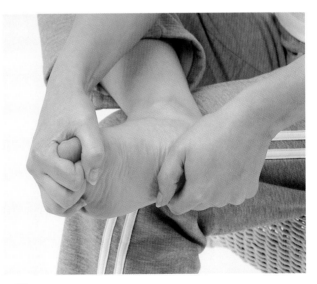

2 Now use the palms of your hands and pads of your fingers to gently stroke all over your foot and ankle. One hand follows the other to create an almost hypnotic wavelike movement. Continue for as long as you wish.

3 Support your ankle with one hand. Make a loosely clenched fist with your free hand and very gently and slowly tap your foot, using the flats of your fingers and heel of your hand. Change hands, as necessary, to cover your whole foot—top and sole.

5 Support your foot or ankle with one hand. Use the other hand to grasp all 5 toes. Your fingers rest on top of your toes with your palm beneath. Now gently bend, stretch, and rotate all 5 toes at once. Repeat 6 times in each direction.

6 Next work on the sole of the foot. Support your foot with one hand. Make a loose fist with your free hand, and use your knuckles to gently knead all around the sole of your foot. Work into those areas of tension, and enjoy the tingling sensation this brings. →

program9   Soothe your feet...continued

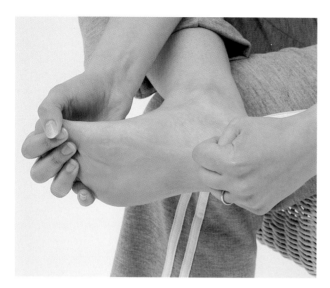

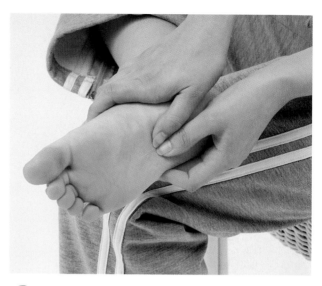

7 Holding your foot with one hand, place the knuckles of the other hand just under the ball of the foot. Stroke your fist firmly and slowly down the sole toward the heel. Feel a releasing stretch under your foot. In the same position as in Step 6, use the heel of your free hand to make a firm, circular movement around the arch of your foot. Make 3 generous circles, keeping your hand soft and relaxed, molding to the shape of your foot.

8 Support your foot in both hands, fingers on top and thumbs on the sole. Press with the pads of your thumbs and, in one long, sweeping stroke, push them upward to the base of the toes and then fan outward to the sides of your foot. Lightly glide over the skin to return to starting point. Repeat 4 times.

WARNING
If you have any conditions that affect your feet, such as arthritis, gout, or diabetes, always check with your physician before carrying out these steps.

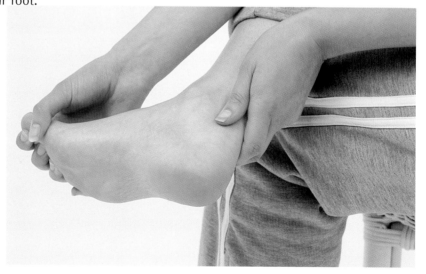

11 In the same position as the previous step, bring your free hand up to your Achilles tendon and continue these gentle circular movements with your palm. Continue as long as you wish.

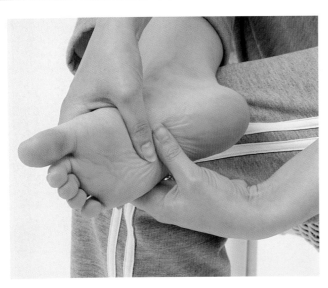

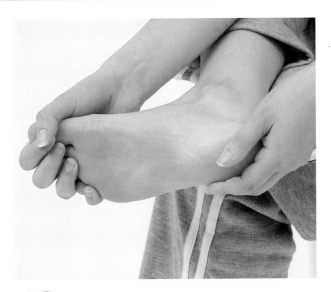

9 With hands held in the same position as Step 8, place one thumb slightly above the other. Now slide your thumbs out toward the sides of the feet and back in toward each other. Continue this crisscross action, working from the base of the heel and back again until the whole of the sole is covered.

10 Supporting your foot or ankle with one hand, cup your heel in the palm of your other hand. Use your palm to make a circular movement around your heel. Keep your hand soft and molded to the shape of the heel and maintain contact.

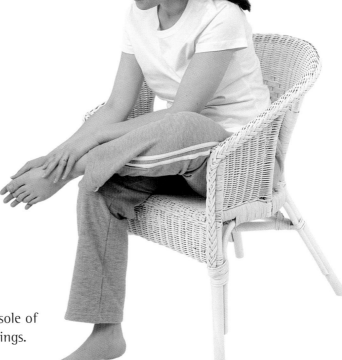

12 Finish the sequence with gentle featherlike strokes all over the top and sole of your foot. Sense the inner peace this brings.

Whenever you take part in a strenuous activity, it is essential that your joints are mobilized and that your muscles are slowly stretched and warmed before you begin. If you are fully prepared, there may be less risk of soreness or injury. Equally vital is a cooldown to allow your body to return gradually to its resting state. These 14 stretches take about 10 minutes and are suitable for a warm-up or cooldown. Stand with your feet hip-width apart and knees relaxed. Move into the stretches gradually, without jerking, and stop if you feel any discomfort. Never force a stretch. Begin gently, and then gradually build up to a more strenuous pace.

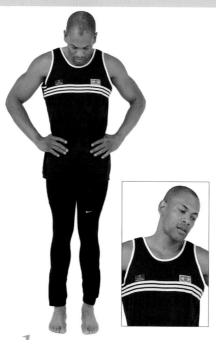

1 Start by warming up your neck muscles. Place your hands on your hips. Now drop your head gently to one side, then to the front and across your chest to the other side. Repeat 3 times, ensuring that the movement is slow and controlled.

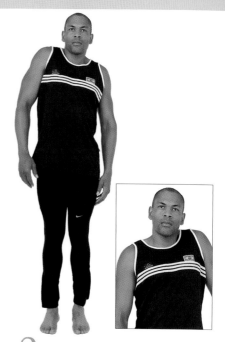

2 With your body facing forward and arms by your sides, circle your shoulders. Begin by pushing one shoulder forward and the other back. Then roll them in a continuous, flowing motion for about 30 seconds. Reverse the direction and repeat the shoulder-rolling action.

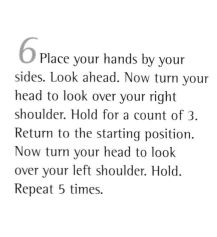

6 Place your hands by your sides. Look ahead. Now turn your head to look over your right shoulder. Hold for a count of 3. Return to the starting position. Now turn your head to look over your left shoulder. Hold. Repeat 5 times.

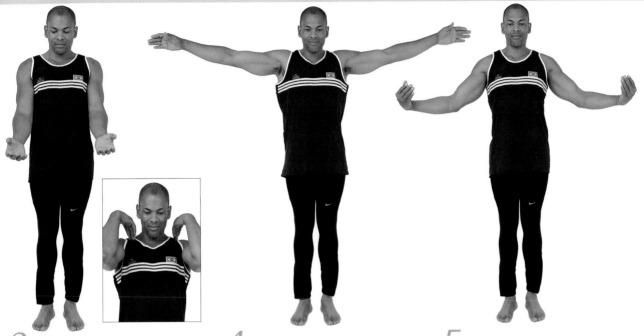

3 Stretch your arms in front of you. Bend your elbows so your hands touch your shoulders. Now straighten your arms with palms facing upward. Repeat 10 times.

4 Place your arms so they are straight out from your sides. Slowly move your arms in increasing circles. Continue for about 30 seconds. Bring your arms to your sides and repeat in the opposite direction.

5 With your arms still outstretched, circle your wrists in a counterclockwise direction. Keep your movements slow and deliberate. Repeat 5 times. Now repeat in the opposite direction.

7 Place your hands on your waist. Now bend your body to the side, allowing a lovely stretch along the other side of the waist. Pull in your abdomen and try not to lean backward or forward. Hold for a count of 5. Return to the starting position and repeat on the other side. ➜

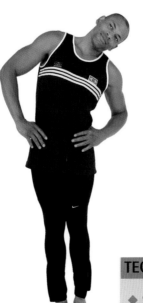

TECHNIQUE CHECKLIST

◆ Stretching   (see pages 38–55)

program 10

Prepare for action...continued

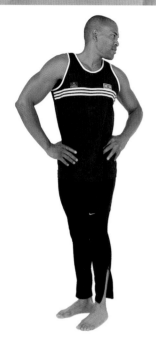

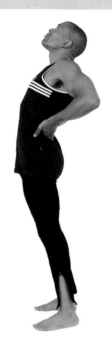

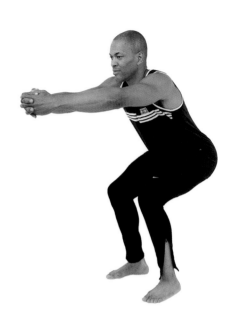

8 Place your hands on your hips. Relax your knees and twist the upper half of your body to the left. Keep your head in line with your upper body. Enjoy the stretch. Hold for a count of 5. Slowly return to the upright position and repeat on the other side.

9 Bring your palms to your lower back. Now lean your upper body back, taking care not to overstretch your neck. Hold for a count of 5. Repeat 3 times. This is a wonderful stretch for shoulder, back, and hip muscles.

10 To loosen hip and leg muscles, try some squats. Stand with your knees bent and feet shoulder-width apart. Keeping your heels flat on the ground, squat as low as you comfortably can. Do not overstretch. Place your hands in front of you to help with balance. Hold for a count of 5 and repeat 3 times.

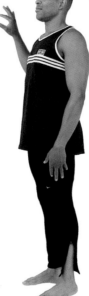

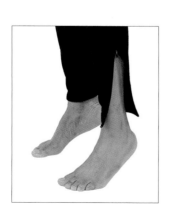

13 Standing with feet shoulder-width apart, raise your heels from the ground, and then lower. Repeat 5 times to exercise your calf muscles.

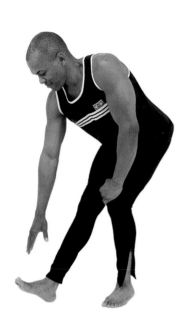

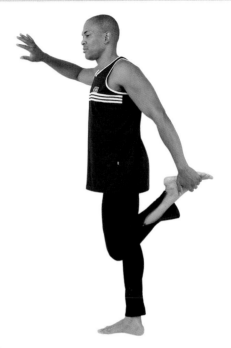

11 This helps stretch and loosen the hamstring muscles at the backs of your thighs. Stand with your right leg a little way in front of your left leg. Your front leg is straight, and your back leg is bent and weight bearing. Place your left hand on your left knee. Lean forward until you feel a pleasant stretch in the back of the thigh. Do not overstretch. Hold for a count of 10. Repeat on the other leg.

12 Now stretch the quadriceps muscle at the front of your thigh. Bend your left leg and bring your foot as far toward your buttocks as is comfortable. Relax your right leg. Grasp your foot or ankle with your left hand. Keep your knees together and hips facing forward. Try not to arch your lower back. Feel the releasing stretch at the front of your thigh. Do not overstretch. Hold for a count of 10. Repeat on the other leg.

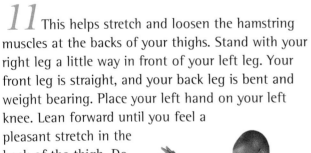

14 Finally, raise one leg from the ground and stretch it in front of you. Now, in a slow and controlled movement, trace the letters of your name with your foot. This is a fun alternative to ankle-circling to help loosen your ankle and foot. Repeat with the other leg.

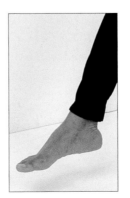

WARNING

It is a good idea to use a chair or wall for support when doing the final steps in this sequence.

Index

Note: Page reference in italic indicates annotated illustration.

(continued)

AUTHOR'S ACKNOWLEDGMENTS

This book has been a real team effort. One daughter Lizi helped put together some of the massage sequences, while the other, Emma, modeled the techniques section. And husband, Richard, acted as a constant source of support and encouragement to us all. Grateful thanks also to Adam, the mirror man. My appreciation to my editor, Richard Emerson, whose sense of humor made even the most tedious tasks uplifting. And of course, my thanks to my agent, Chelsey Fox, and to Cindy, Georgina, Geoff, and Gavin, who make working within the Cico team such a privilege.

PUBLISHER'S ACKNOWLEDGMENTS

The Publishers would like to thank Corinne Roberts and Kate Strutt for modeling. Thanks also go to the Pier for supply of props.